American Medical Association
Physicians dedicated to the health of America

# Twelve Steps to a

# Carefree Retirement

## How to Avoid Preretirement Anxiety Syndrome

**Paul H. Sutherland** CFP

# Twelve Steps to a Carefree Retirement
## How to Avoid Preretirement Anxiety Syndrome

Internet address: http://www.ama-assn.org

Information contained in this publication does not constitute legal
or business advice and should not be substituted for the independent
advice of an attorney or business consultant. Opinions expressed
in this publication are not necessarily those of the AMA.

Additional copies of this book may be ordered from the
American Medical Association. For order information,
call toll-free 800 621-8335. Mention product number OP208399.

ISBN 0-89970-995-8

BP37:99-0189:3.3M:8/99

Dedicated to all the
Grandmas and Granddads
who hug their grandchildren,
listen to their children,
smile, and love life.

# About the Author

**Paul H. Sutherland, CFP, MBA,** is president and founder of Financial & Investment Management Group of Suttons Bay, Michigan, and Maui, Hawaii. Financial & Investment Management Group is SEC registered as an Investment Advisor. This advice-driven firm is structured as fee-only, meaning they receive no transaction-related compensation or commissions.

Paul received his MBA from Lake Superior State University, is a Certified Financial Planner, and is a member in good standing of the National Association of Personal Financial Advisors. He has also completed the College of Financial Planning's Advanced Studies Course: Investment Strategies and Portfolio Management. His range of expertise includes financial planning, portfolio management and construction, conscientious investments, and mutual funds.

Individuals and corporations from across the United States have sought Paul's advice concerning such issues as estate and tax planning, retirement, and financial and investment management. He is in demand as a speaker, having given presentations to the Kansas Medical Society, World Future Society, Baylor College of Medicine, Northwestern Michigan Osteopathic Physicians Association, and Northwestern Michigan Association of CPAs, among others.

Paul is the author of three previously published books. *Financial Strategies for Physicians* (W.B. Saunders of Harcourt Brace Jovanovich) and *Physician's Financial Sourcebook* (Financial Sourcebook Publishing) were published in 1987 and 1998, respectively. His latest book, *Zenvesting: The Art of Abundance & Managing Money,* also published by Financial Sourcebook Publishing, was released in November 1998. *Twelve Steps to a Carefree Retirement* is his first publishing venture with the American Medical Association.

Over the past twenty years Paul has been a contributing editor and/or writer for many journals and magazines, including *Dental Management, Business Ethics, National Psychologist, Financial Planner, Physicians Management,* and *Publishing Entrepreneur.* He has been interviewed by *Barron's, The Wall Street Journal, Wall Street Transcript,* and *Money Magazine,* and has appeared on the local NBC affiliate's *Money Watch* program.

# Foreword

Retirement! Retirement!

In all my years as a financial planner and money manager to physicians, I can't remember ever having had a financial planning goal session with a physician client where retirement security was not a top priority. Physicians are highly skilled, self-reliant professionals; but often, as they approach retirement, the idea of being financially dependent on a portfolio of investments is a very unnerving proposition. They simply don't realize until too late in their careers how difficult it is to make informed and educated decisions regarding retirement.

Setting retirement goals is easy; but actual retirement is an emotional, physical, and intellectual challenge for all but the most prepared physicians.

I have designed this book to place you in the "most prepared" category. The steps involving budgeting, tax issues, risk management, saving, and investing are the easy part of retirement. Much more troublesome retirement concerns have to do with questions like "What will I do?" "Will I feel worthless?" and many other normal, very real fears.

This book will help you throughout your career, culminating in a happy, successful retirement. I define retirement as "the ability to live, relax, and enjoy life dependent on a well-constructed retirement plan." My editor thought I should add that "a successful retirement requires a lengthy list of avocations and goals with plenty of opportunity to pursue them."

Everyone has a different idea of retirement. One couple may wish to bicycle around the world, then go on to a second career, while another may simply plan to relax, read a long list of literary classics, and play golf twice a week. Regardless of the activities planned or retirement envisioned, what I do realize is just how important a successful retirement plan is to physicians.

I also have a great deal of respect for physicians who choose not to retire— ever. This choice shows that some physicians have created a working environment so pleasurable and a career so fulfilling that retirement has no allure.

I firmly believe you can have it all: a successful career followed by a full retirement with ample time for family, friends, and your own physical, mental, and spiritual needs. This book will show you how to do that.

# Acknowledgments

"I'd love to write a book for you about retirement," I blurted out to Suzanne Fraker, AMA Senior Acquisitions Editor, at about the same time I was putting the final touches on *Physician's Financial Sourcebook*, another recent book project. You are holding the fruits of that conversation with Suzanne. Thanks to Suzanne for the support and diligent help I received from her and her colleagues: my editor Jean Roberts, communications coordinator Rosalyn Carlton, print coordinator Don Frye, and marketing manager Patrick Dati, all of the AMA, and designer Steve Straus, all of whom helped make *Twelve Steps to a Carefree Retirement* a reality.

I wish to thank past AMA presidents Edward Annis and Anne Barlow, James Burrus, Stephen Ward, and others who shared their stories with us and provided input on what they felt should and must be addressed in a book for physicians on retirement.

This is the third book project where my brother Matt has served as my chief editor-cowriter-interviewer. Matt is a committed perfectionist, able to take my scribbles and words and turn them into clearly stated concepts that can be easily understood by those without the business education, training, and experience that I have been immersed in throughout my career. We spent a number of weekends gulping strong coffee in an effort to meet Suzanne and Jean's deadlines. I wish to thank my loving wife, Kim, and sister-in-law, Victoria, for their support of Matt and me, as we missed a few "family Saturday gigs" in order to complete this project.

This project was over a year in the making, during which time I asked for input from many of my clients on what they felt should be included in the book. They shared personal retirement stories, often with tears in their eyes, to help make *Twelve Steps to a Carefree Retirement* more than simply a book of numbers and strategies. For confidentiality reasons, I am unable to list them by name, but they know how deeply I appreciate their input.

Noah Creamer of Arc Technologies was my "puter" man (as my four-year-old calls him). He installed the high-powered voice recognition system that allowed me to export text electronically to our office network and greatly expedite the writing and editing process. Without him, this book would still be a dream.

As always, incredible help came from Linda Brzezinski (who has typed manuscripts and articles for me since 1980) and another of our patient staff, Sandy Erickson, who worked extra hours and helped Matt decipher my scribbles.

My need to work on this project put greater pressure on each of my business colleagues as they added to their schedules to free up my time as the manager of a hundred million dollar plus investment management and financial planning firm. Thanks to Robin Bahle, Matt Bohrer, Mike Pippin (president of Pension Service Design, Inc), Julie Webber, Alice Vanni, Barb Thoms, and Barb McClellan.

More weekends and evenings were worked by my colleague, Barry A. Hyman, keeping careful watch over our client portfolios throughout these recent, very volatile months of 1998–1999.

Finally, thanks to all the "philosophers and thinkers" I have known—through their spoken words and writings—who have taught me that life is more than money.

I unscientifically queried a number of fee-only financial advisors who work with physicians and used my own practice to come up with the informal ranges and statistics found in many of the sidebars that begin with "The average fee-only financial advisor serving physicians found that . . ."

Special thanks to Kate Thornhill, CPA; Jack Niederhofer, CPA, CFP; Bert Whitehead, LLD, CFP; Marge Schiller, CPA; Mitchell J. Metz, CFP; Lawrence Howes; Scott Neal, CPA; and David Foster, CPA, CFP.

# Disclaimer

Advice given in this book is general in nature and may not pertain to your specific needs. If you have any doubt whether the information contained herein pertains to your situation, you should seek competent financial planning advice.

Mutual funds and companies listed in this book are not necessarily endorsed by the author, editor, or publisher of *Twelve Steps to a Carefree Retirement*. Inflation, taxation, and a host of new investment and tax law changes occur almost daily. The reader's responsibility is to assess the risk or appropriateness of any investment or strategy on their own behalf.

Our goal is to provide the most objective and purposeful information possible. We believe there is no substitute for integrity when it comes to serving our readers. We expect a degree of criticism based on our sharp commentary on commissioned salespeople, ie, stockbrokers selling load and commissionable mutual funds, insurance agents pushing insurance products for large commissions, and inept, unqualified people with little experience giving financial advice.

If you have any questions or comments on any of the information in this book, please contact us so that we can review your comments with other professionals and respond. In addition, if you have information you wish to see in future editions of this book, please feel free to write us at PO Box 40, 417 St. Joseph Street, Suttons Bay, MI 49682; e-mail us at pub@fimg.net; or phone us at 800 632-5528 or 616 271-3915.

It is our sincere hope that those who read this book will achieve greater financial security—with less risk—and live a happy and balanced life.

# Table of Contents

About the Author                                                                iv

Foreword                                                                         v

Acknowledgments                                                                  vi

Disclaimer                                                                       viii


chapter one        Quantify Your Retirement Income Needs                         1

chapter two        Manage Your Debt                                             17

chapter three      Carefully Insure Yourself Against Risk and Misfortune        25

chapter four       Control Taxes                                               37

chapter five       Save                                                        45

chapter six        Retirement Plans                                            57

chapter seven      Invest Wisely                                               71

chapter eight      Do-It-Yourself Portfolio Management                         81

chapter nine       Dollar-Cost-Averaging                                      107

chapter ten        Once Retired, Plan to Live Forever                         117

chapter eleven     Monitor Your Progress: Straight Talk on Growing Old        127

chapter twelve     The Money Is Easy                                          133

chapter thirteen   Estate Planning                                            141


Glossary                                                                      149

Appendix           Investor Resources                                         169

Index                                                                         185

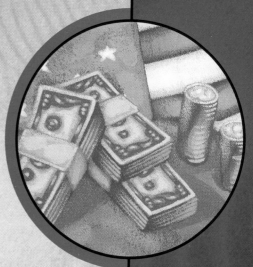

# chapter one

# Quantify Your Retirement Income Needs

**P**ause and think about what your first day of retirement will be like. Will you pack for a trip? Will you spend the day looking for a new home? What about your first week? First month? Year? Will you spend several months traveling? Will you work part-time—not so much for the money, but for the feeling of worth you get from helping others? Will you reengineer yourself for a new career? Think hard about these questions so you can quantify how much you'll need to support your lifestyle in a relaxing and comfortable retirement.

Amazingly, some retired physicians have busier schedules outlined in their Franklin Planners than they did before retirement. Tee time with men's league at 6 AM; breakfast with wife at 10 AM; mentor with residents from 11:00 to 1:00; lunch with former partner (call first) at 1:00; tennis with wife (doubles) 2:30 to 4:30; dinner;

> **The average fee-only financial advisor serving physicians found that ...**
> A goal of their average young physician client is to be able to retire between the ages of fifty and sixty-five.

then baby-sit kid's kids. Others get up in the morning and say, "I've got a feeling that the steelhead trout are running today," and roll their eyes at their Franklin Planner cohorts. Everyone's retirement is different; the goal is to make sure that you achieve whichever retirement vision you have for yourself. This chapter will help you quantify what your retirement income needs will be and how much money you'll need to retire comfortably.

Your first job is to visualize your ideal retirement lifestyle. With the help of your spouse (or significant other), fantasize about the wildest, most creative, outrageous, and coolest retirement you can imagine. Write it all down— every fantasy, every whim, every excursion. Then set it aside for awhile, think about it, discuss it a bit, then start to solidify a more permanent image. You *can* have it all in retirement, including the freedom to relax and enjoy life. To feel and savor life. To experience life's many colors, sounds, and textures. The wonderful perspective of age and experience gives us this opportunity in retirement. We are more qualified to identify and embrace the beauty around us. The opportunity may be much the same that we had while we were working, but we were too busy then and unwilling to break out of our routines. Retirement grants us the time to do so.

The reality is that your retirement adventure will change over time. Often retirees (Don't you hate that word?) will find that their lives are very busy and full of activity early in their retirement adventure; later, this dizzying busyness wanes until a happy medium is reached. Keep this in mind as you fill out the Retirement Worksheet (see Figure 1.1). I have noticed a pretty even split between clients who engaged in very busy early retirement years, slowing down as they got older, spending more time with children, close friends, a good book, surfing the Net, and other more passive activities, and others who have become much busier over time. One eighty-three-year-old client reported, "My wife isn't happy unless we always have three different vacations planned, scheduled, and paid for." I remember taking an early morning walk one beautiful Maui morning and almost being run over by a near-centenarian biker peddling his way up to the Haleakala mountain summit.

Retirement lasts a long time, but it doesn't feel that way psychologically because as we age, time shrinks. When you were ten years old, one year was one-tenth of your life, while when you are seventy, that year is only one-seventieth of your life. It will feel like it passes seven times faster than the years of your youth. Realize when filling out the upcoming worksheets that you will have ample time, and that time will have a different meaning to you than it has in the past, both because you're older (more understanding) and because each day in retirement will seem shorter.

Thus, if your desire is to travel in retirement, plan on your trips being longer, more leisurely, less hectic than trips you take today. "Know yourself" when using age as a determinant of future activity level, mental capacity, vitality, etc. Some people are old at thirty, while others remain young at ninety. Not to belabor this point, but if you think you'll be old at seventy, then you can count on being old at seventy.

# Quantify Retirement Income Needs

Step 2 of the process is to quantify what your retirement lifestyle will cost in today's dollars. Do not fret about inflation or deflation when completing step 2 of the Retirement Worksheet. In other words, don't say gas will cost $5.00 a gallon or that cars will cost $100,000. Use numbers as if you were retiring today. (It is your portfolio's job to ensure that you'll have enough at retirement. Simply be as reasonable and exact as you can in completing your Realistic/Fantasy Retirement Budget.

**The average fee-only financial advisor serving physicians found that . . .** A goal of their average physician client is to retire with an annual income of $100,000 to $250,000 in "today's" dollars.

From my experience, the main budget buster in retirement is the needs (wants) of children and grandchildren. If it is your desire to help your children with your retirement savings, then by all means include the amount you wish to use to help them in your budget. The worksheet allows a little wriggle room to help ensure that you can stay retired and within your budget should unforeseen expenses come up. However, be aware that if you have trouble saying no to your children before retirement, you'll have trouble saying no in retirement.

# Consider Long-Term Care

I have found that when one or both retired spouses require long-term care or a nursing home, budget expenses actually go down. Traveling and many other activities are restrained due to the sickness or injury, and the well spouse spends much of his or her time caring for the loved one. If the expenses in your budget for travel/vacations, entertainment, sanity, fun, personal development, and insurance/health total more than $30,000, then it is probably unnecessary to have special provisions in place for long-term care. Your monthly budget should assume at least $250 per month per person for normal insurance/health care needs.

# Estimate Income from Other Sources

Step 3 asks you to carry your estimate of total income needs from step 2 over to the first box on the step 3 worksheet. Assuming Social Security is still viable, that amount should be included in any retirement projection; however, never assume Social Security will be over one-fourth of your income just in case the program is not completely solvent. In retirement planning, look at Social Security income as gravy.

If you or your spouse qualify for a fixed pension, naturally this income should be added to and considered in step 3. Estimate the pension income assuming a Joint and 100 Percent Survivor benefit. Do not assume anything other than that unless you are working with a competent fee-only retirement planner. Some insurance agents will push life insurance products designed to allow you to take a Joint and 0 Percent Survivor benefit so you allegedly end up with more income in retirement. I find these schemes, often called "retirement enhancers" or "benefit guaranteed plans," do not work well; they are not worth the risk. If you consider such plans, get everything in writing from the insurance company's home office, not just from the commissioned salesperson.

# Answer the "How Much Will I Need" Question

Step 4 brings it all together in the process of quantifying your retirement nest egg needs. Of course, you will still have liquidity/emergency funds safely invested in a cash management account. And while at retirement you may not pay off all your debts, you need to assume that you will. This may entail calling your banker to see how much you will owe at retirement. If you decide on a second home, you will need to quantify that need and list it in step 4.

For many, the first item of retirement business is to take an extravagant, once-in-a-lifetime vacation, including all the children and grandchildren, to celebrate retirement. Some retirees do not distinguish between what is considered a vacation and normal retirement lifestyle. For example, one of my successfully retired clients and his wife spend three months a year at their cottage (home) on an island in northern Michigan, one month at a condo time share in the Caribbean, and a fair amount of the balance of the year at their real (so to speak, especially for tax purposes) home in Nevada. They do not consider the time spent in Michigan or the Caribbean as vacations but rather as part of their retirement lifestyle. Retirees tend to settle into a consistent lifestyle (as well as a consistent yearly budget), so special provisions must be made only for that one-of-a-kind dream vacation.

# Answer the "How Much for How Much" Question

How much income can you comfortably draw from a portfolio to support your retirement lifestyle? The answer to this question depends on many factors since the future is unknown and all available information is basically incomplete; approximations are as close as we can get to an answer. Historically, the stock market has beat inflation by 7 percent to 9 percent per year over very long periods of time. Over shorter periods—during crashes and bear markets—the stock market has significantly underperformed inflation, and the stock market's volatility has dashed the retirement hopes of many investors. Bonds—even government bonds, the seeming bastion of safety—performed horribly during the inflationary 1970s but turned around wonderfully as inflation came under control in the 1980s. Money market investments, while providing predictability of principal and considerable safety and stability, have barely kept pace with inflation over the years. Real estate and similar investments, like gold, silver, oil, and art, also seem to be controlled by the whims of cycles, manias, and world economic events.

Depending on the prevailing cycle, it can sometimes seem that investing is an impossible task, while at other times everything turns out to be a winner. Further complicating the matter of managing portfolios in retirement is that, once retired, you are wholly dependent on your portfolio and not your skills for income. At retirement it is easy to become obsessed about your portfolio and its ability to comfortably, safely, and reliably provide you with lifetime income security. The best assurance that you will have plenty at retirement is to have plenty at retirement.

How much can you comfortably draw on your retirement portfolio? The answer to this question depends on your risk tolerance and portfolio constraints. If you are long-term oriented, understand financial markets, emphasize investments that are undervalued, and look at your money as a tool, then you can draw up to 6 percent per year on your portfolio. If you are short-term-capital-preservation oriented, don't like any volatility to your portfolio, and would lose sleep if your portfolio lost over 5 percent of its value, then 3 percent per year is probably the income constraint you should place on your portfolio. At one end of the spectrum is the more aggressive investor, drawing $60,000 per year from a $1 million dollar portfolio, while at the other is the conservative investor, looking at no more than $30,000 per year from a $1 million portfolio. Figure 1.2 (Managing Your Portfolio Like You'll Live Forever) lists the lump sum needed to provide income at various risk constraints. Use it to complete step 5 of the worksheet. Future chapters will discuss how portfolios should be managed to ensure that your money is working for you consistent with your needs, desires, and risk tolerance.

We will now take a long, hard look at your assets, liabilities, income, and expenses because financial retirement success is about being efficient in the way you spend and save, as well as knowing the reality of your life. The Assets and Liabilities Worksheet (Figure 1.3) will help you more clearly understand your financial reality. What is your biggest financial asset? Your skills—not your home, your retirement plan, your office buildings, or your stocks. It's your skills, your ability to earn lots of income.

Fill out the form, including the section on goals, as we will use this information in future chapters. Some sample goals are listed below to help you define yours:

- Build net worth
- Tax efficiency
- Build investment portfolio
- Financial direction
- Increase investment returns
- Finance education
- Increase charitable donations
- Debt management
- Travel
- Build emergency fund
- Retirement security
- Reduce estate settlement cost
- Build an efficient insurance program
- Confidentiality planning
- Review investment portfolio
- Make work enjoyable
- Work less
- Family financial security

**Figure 1.1**

# Retirement Worksheet

## Step 1

Describe your ideal retirement lifestyle:

_____

_____

_____

_____

_____

_____

*Coaching:* Two homes or one main home and travel, travel two months in winter/summer, second career, charitable pursuits, educational pursuits.

Describe your ideal retirement lifestyle in years 2 to 5:

_____

_____

_____

_____

_____

Describe your ideal retirement lifestyle in years 5 to 10:

_____

_____

_____

_____

_____

**Figure 1.1** *continued*

Describe your ideal retirement lifestyle in years 10 to 20:

_____

_____

_____

_____

_____

Describe your ideal retirement lifestyle in years 20 to 30:

_____

_____

_____

_____

_____

Describe your ideal retirement lifestyle in years 30 and beyond:

_____

_____

_____

_____

_____

## Figure 1.1 *continued*

### Step 2

Quantify your retirement lifestyle costs in today's dollars.

| Realistic Fantasy Retirement Budget | Annual Estimate | | Monthly Estimate |
|---|---|---|---|
| Home maintenance (estimate 2% of value) | $_____ | ÷ 12 = | $_____ |
| Second home maintenance (estimate 2% of value) | $_____ | ÷ 12 = | $_____ |
| Travel/Vacations | $_____ | ÷ 12 = | $_____ |
| Home insurance | $_____ | ÷ 12 = | $_____ |
| Property taxes | $_____ | ÷ 12 = | $_____ |
| Car payments* | $_____ | ÷ 12 = | $_____ |
| Auto expenses | $_____ | ÷ 12 = | $_____ |
| Phone | $_____ | ÷ 12 = | $_____ |
| Electricity/Heating | $_____ | ÷ 12 = | $_____ |
| Food | $_____ | ÷ 12 = | $_____ |
| Entertainment (nonvacation, eg, movies, plays, dinners) | $_____ | ÷ 12 = | $_____ |
| Subscriptions/Computer expenses | $_____ | ÷ 12 = | $_____ |
| Sanity (eg, yoga, counseling) | $_____ | ÷ 12 = | $_____ |
| Fun (eg, wine, cigars, latte) | $_____ | ÷ 12 = | $_____ |
| Personal development/education | $_____ | ÷ 12 = | $_____ |
| Helping others | $_____ | ÷ 12 = | $_____ |
| Tithing | $_____ | ÷ 12 = | $_____ |
| Insurance/Health | $_____ | ÷ 12 = | $_____ |
| Helping children/grandchildren | $_____ | ÷ 12 = | $_____ |
| **Total annual/monthly expenses estimated at** | | | $_____ |
| Plus 65% to estimate expenses for taxes and divine surplus | $_____ | ÷ 12 = | $_____ |
| **Equals total annual/monthly income needed estimated at** | $_____ | ÷ 12 = | $_____ |

\* You'll pay cash for cars in retirement but will need to budget for them based on your needs. For example, if you plan to replace your $36,000 car every three years, you will need to put $1,000 aside monthly as your car payment.

*Note:* This exercise should be done with your spouse.

**Figure 1.1** *continued*

## Step 3

Estimate income needed from portfolio.

|  | Annual |
|---|---|
| Estimate of total income needs from last line of step 2 | $ _____ |
| Less estimated Social Security income* | – $ _____ |
| Less income from fixed pension, etc | – $ _____ |
| **Equals total income needed from portfolio** | = $ _____ |

\* If both you and your spouse work and earn over $50,000 each, estimate Social Security annual income as follows:
Retired at 50 = $ 9,000
Retired at 55 = $10,000
Retired at 60 = $12,000
Retired at 65 = $18,000

If just one spouse worked, estimate Social Security annual income as follows:
Retired at 50 = $ 6,000
Retired at 55 = $ 7,000
Retired at 60 = $ 9,000
Retired at 65 = $10,000

## Step 4

Quantify your lump sum need for a "you'll live forever" retirement portfolio.

The percent of income you can comfortably draw upon from your portfolio will depend on your risk tolerance as described below and in future chapters. Take your monthly income needs and divide the total sum by the following factors:

| | |
|---|---|
| Aggressive investor—long-term equity income oriented | .05% |
| Balanced investor—long-term total return oriented | .045% |
| Yield income investor/bond/income stocks oriented | .04% |
| Capital preservation money market and bond investor | .03% |

Recommended maximum percentage to draw on investment portfolio in retirement:

| Volatility Constraint | Percent to Draw Annually | Percent to Draw Monthly | $1 million = Income of Annually | Monthly |
|---|---|---|---|---|
| 35%, aggressive investor | 6.0% | .05% | $60,000 | $5,000 |
| 25%, balanced investor | 5.4 | .045 | 54,000 | 4,500 |
| 15%, yield investor | 4.8 | .04 | 48,000 | 4,000 |
| 5%, capital preservation | 3.6 | .03 | 36,000 | 3,000 |

---

## Figure 1.1 *continued*

If you're a balanced investor and need an income of $160,000 annually, you'll need to divide $160,000 by 5.4%, which means you'll need $2,962,963 to provide you with an annual income of $160,000.

(Portfolio income need equals balance from step 3 divided by your annual percentage to withdraw from above, which will in turn equal the lump sum you need to retire.)

*Note:* Figure 1.1 helps do this work for you.

## Step 5

Quantify your total investment needs

*Note:* Generally you'll be completely debt-free at retirement, having paid off all debts before then. If not, you'll need to anticipate the lump sum needed for these debts and add them to the lump sum you need to retire. It is OK to have debts at retirement; there actually can be advantages to it via tax savings, etc; but to make your projections work, we must turn debts into lump sums.

| | |
|---|---|
| Lump sum of six months' budget/liquidity needs (half of total annual need from step 2) | $_____ |
| Lump sum to pay off debts on home, car, etc | $_____ |
| Lump sum for second home | $_____ |
| Lump sum for boat, dream vacation, etc | $_____ |
| Lump sum for retirement income needs* | $_____ |
| **Total liquid investment/income assets needed to retire** | $_____ |

* Future chapters will help you build a plan to achieve this lump sum need. Don't worry about this big number right now; savings, time, and compound returns will get you there.

## Figure 1.2

# Managing Your Portfolio Like You'll Live Forever

| Annual Income Needed | Lump Sum Needed for Retirement Income | | | |
|---|---|---|---|---|
| | Aggressive | Balanced | Yield | Capital Preservation |
| $ 50,000 | $ 833,333.33 | $ 925,925.93 | $ 1,041,666.67 | $ 1,388,888.89 |
| 75,000 | 1,250,000.00 | 1,388,888.89 | 1,562,500.00 | 2,083,333.33 |
| 100,000 | 1,666,666.67 | 1,851,851.85 | 2,083,333.33 | 2,777,777.78 |
| 125,000 | 2,083,333.33 | 2,314,814.81 | 2,604,166.67 | 3,472,222.22 |
| 150,000 | 2,500,000.00 | 2,777,777.78 | 3,125,000.00 | 4,166,666.67 |
| 175,000 | 2,916,666.67 | 3,240,740.74 | 3,645,833.33 | 4,861,111.11 |
| 200,000 | 3,333,333.33 | 3,703,703.70 | 4,166,666.67 | 5,555,555.56 |
| 225,000 | 3,750,000.00 | 4,166,666.67 | 4,687,500.00 | 6,250,000.00 |
| 250,000 | 4,166,666.67 | 4,629,629.63 | 5,208,333.33 | 6,944,444.44 |
| 300,000 | 5,000,000.00 | 5,555,555.56 | 6,250,000.00 | 8,333,333.33 |
| 350,000 | 5,833,333.33 | 6,481,481.48 | 7,291,666.67 | 9,722,222.22 |
| 400,000 | 6,666,666.67 | 7,407,407.41 | 8,333,333.33 | 11,111,111.11 |
| 450,000 | 7,500,000.00 | 8,333,333.33 | 9,375,000.00 | 12,500,000.00 |
| 600,000 | 10,000,000.00 | 11,111,111.11 | 12,500,000.00 | 16,666,666.67 |
| 700,000 | 11,666,666.67 | 12,962,962.96 | 14,583,333.33 | 19,444,444.44 |

*Note:* Naturally, the future is unknown, as are future returns on assets. The above is a "best guess" analysis of reasonable returns to expect to keep you retired. The main risk is your long-term portfolio results and the effects of inflation/deflation on your income needs and portfolio. This table assumes your portfolio principal will grow and your income will increase over the years to help offset inflation.

**Figure 1.3**

# Financial Information:
# Assets and Liabilities Worksheet

## Assets

**Investments/Liquid Assets**

Checking/Cash $_____

Money Market funds $_____

**Other Investments**

_____ $_____

_____ $_____

_____ $_____

_____ $_____

**Retirement Plans**

_____ $_____

_____ $_____

_____ $_____

_____ $_____

**Other Personal Assets**

Personal residence 1 $_____
(Cost $_____)

Personal residence 2 $_____
(Cost $_____)

Furniture, appliances, jewelry, $_____
art, etc

Life insurance $_____

_____ $_____

Automobile(s) $_____

_____ $_____

Other _____ $_____

_____ $_____

**Figure 1.3** *continued*

**Business Assets**

Checking/Cash             $_____

Money Market funds      $_____

Real assets                $_____

_____    $_____

Goodwill value           $_____

**Total Assets**             $_____

## Liabilities

**Home Mortgage**

Monthly payment    $_____
Balance                   $_____
Balloon year_____
Interest rate_____%

Monthly payment    $_____
Balance                   $_____
Balloon year_____
Interest rate_____%

Monthly payment    $_____
Balance                   $_____
Balloon year_____
Interest rate_____%

Monthly payment    $_____
Balance                   $_____
Balloon year_____
Interest rate_____%

Monthly payment    $_____

Balance                   $_____

Other Liabilities

_____    $_____

_____    $_____

**Total Liabilities**        $_____

**Net Worth**            $_____
(Total Assets – Total Liabilities)

**Figure 1.3** *continued*

## Income

| Prior years | Amount | Source |
|---|---|---|
| _____ | $_____ | _____ |
| _____ | $_____ | _____ |
| _____ | $_____ | _____ |

| Current year | Estimated amount | Source |
|---|---|---|
| _____ | $_____ | _____ |
| _____ | $_____ | _____ |
| _____ | $_____ | _____ |

**Goals/Notes:**_____

_____

_____

_____

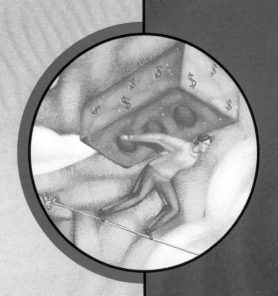

# chapter two

# Manage Your Debt

"**Y**ou can have it all" was the brash proclamation made in the Foreword. But there are conditions attached to having it all, of course—namely, a well-constructed budget and debt management plan. But the *real* key is defining your own sense of reality. And the reality of a successful retirement is that you must balance your work life with your family and personal life. I have yet to work with a physician client whom I felt could not succeed in having a lifestyle profuse with family, vacations, a nice home, and cars, all the while accumulating the necessary assets for a full retirement. By necessity, physicians quickly learn to budget their professional time in a sensible, businesslike manner. These same time management skills (managing appointments, obligations, commitments) are also required to run a family budget.

Creating a budget requires that you fill out the worksheet shown in Figure 2.1 (Monthly Budget Sheet), and then monitor your monthly expenses for a few months so that you get a feel for the flow of money in and out of your household. Most people are prudent about their monthly expenses and tend to live within their means. Budgets are susceptible, however, to financial trauma and unexpected needs, such as children's education, purchase of a new home or office building, an investment with improperly structured debt, etc.

Try to monitor your income and expenses for more than three months to get a picture of normal variations in expenses. For example, summer or winter vacations, tuitions, and such will cause increases, but over several months you should get an accurate average. Once you have done that, calculate your average monthly expenses on the same budget worksheet. At this point, it also might be helpful to look at one or the other of two very good family budgeting software programs: Quicken and Microsoft Money.

Notice on the personal budget worksheet that the amount left to invest (after income tax) is not considered a monthly expense. This is to remind you that your money should make the best use of tax shelters like IRAs, tax-sheltered 403(b) accounts (TSAs), and retirement plan trusts, as well as be tax efficient by using proper business form, which is discussed in later chapters.

It is necessary to write down the amount you paid in income taxes for that three-month period. There is also a place for your total debts and total monthly debt payments. This is because the two areas of budgeting that most often get out of balance are income taxes and debt management.

You will find it inconvenient and difficult to change your monthly fixed expenses other than to rearrange your debt or tax payments. It is rarely beneficial to drastically change your lifestyle while trying to reduce expenses unless you have a very specific goal in mind that is worth the sacrifice.

**Figure 2.1**

# Monthly Budget Sheet

| | Month 1 | Month 2 | Month 3 | Month Average |
|---|---|---|---|---|
| Income Total/Month | | | | |
| Expenses | | | | |
| House/Rent payments | | | | |
| Home insurance | | | | |
| Property taxes | | | | |
| Car payments | | | | |
| Auto expenses | | | | |
| Phone (personal) | | | | |
| Electricity/Heating | | | | |
| Food | | | | |
| Child care | | | | |
| Entertainment | | | | |
| Holiday | | | | |
| Sanity (yoga, counseling) | | | | |
| Fun (wine, cigars, latte) | | | | |
| Personal development | | | | |
| Helping others | | | | |
| Tithing | | | | |
| Insurance (life, health, home) | | | | |
| Second home | | | | |
| Net investment expenses | | | | |
| Home maintenance | | | | |
| Credit cards | | | | |
| Other | | | | |
| **Total Expenses** | | | | |
| (Subtract expenses from income total) | | | | |
| **A**=Total/Month for investment and income tax | | | | |
| **B**=Income tax | | | | |
| Surplus/Deficit Subtract **B** from **A** | | | | |

We will therefore concentrate on proper debt management. Tax management, the other part of budgeting that is commonly out of balance, will be addressed in later chapters. Return to the monthly budget worksheet after you are more experienced in the proper use of tax management, and at that point see what can be done to reduce your tax load, thereby increasing the amount of money you can dedicate to investments and lifestyle.

The key to debt management is to structure your payments over the longest term at the lowest tax-deductible interest rate. Many physicians, especially young physicians, find themselves with large debt payments on short-term loans. This short-term debt, coupled with high taxes and tremendous consumer spending (first home, furniture, car, etc), causes young physicians to be perpetually strapped for cash and anxiety ridden.

It is important to understand that your income will be consistent and significant, and you should therefore manage your debt in a fashion that accounts for the fact that you have a thirty- to forty-year practice life. There is nothing wrong with spreading your payments out over a long period of time. To spread payments out, however, you must trust yourself and use debt only when necessary, whether it is to start up a practice or improve your lifestyle.

Figure 2.2 (Debt Restructuring—New Physician) will help you to decide whether rearranging your debt makes sense. The sample financial plan shows a more holistic example of debt rearrangement than the microscopic view offered by debt management worksheets.

Regardless of the many reasons debt is acquired—experiencing financial trauma, purchasing a home, paying last year's taxes—most people neglect to manage, or even analyze, their debt to find the best way to structure it. Eventually they end up with a mishmash of mismanaged debt that prevents them from achieving their goals.

Keep in mind that the improper use of debt can ruin years of well-laid plans. Especially avoid using debt to make investments that have significant risk or where the income from the investment is targeted to cover the debt payment. For example, if you purchase an apartment complex with a loan that has a debt service of $1,000/month, you should not assume that the income from your project will pay that debt. Be prepared to handle the $1,000 monthly debt service on your own, exclusive of the income from the property. While this approach is very conservative and will upset a few real estate agents, it allows you to avoid accumulating debt service that you cannot completely cover out of your personal service income.

Naturally, whenever you use debt to make an investment, or for any other purpose, you should have adequate disability income insurance. If you were unable to work due to illness or injury, you would have enough income

**Figure 2.2**

# Debt Restructuring— New Physician

| | Value | Loan Amount | Payment |
|---|---|---|---|
| **Current Situation** | | | |
| Home | $550,000 | $380,000 (15 years at 7%) | $3,415 |
| School loan | Priceless | $110,000 | $2,200 |
| Auto | $ 26,000 | $ 25,000 (4 years at 6%) | $ 587 |
| Furniture | $ 22,000 | $ 15,000 (5 years at 5%) | $ 283 |
| Credit cards | Ease | $ 10,000 (10% to 18%) | ? |
| **Totals** | | $540,000 | $6,485 |

*Note:* Need $80,000 cash for liquidity cash needs via second mortgage line of credit, 40lk loan availability, etc.

| | Value | Loan Amount | Payment |
|---|---|---|---|
| **Recommended** | | | |
| Home | $550,000 | $440,000 | $3,077 |
| Home | Second mortgage | 110,000 | 1,100 |
| **Totals** | | $550,000 | $4,177 |

*Note:* Local bank granted line of credit at $70,000 on signature and assignment of life insurance.

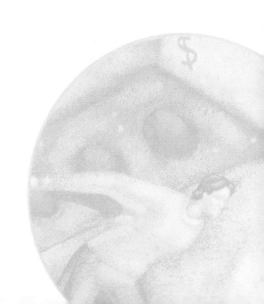

from your disability policy to pay your debt service, while providing an income to maintain your lifestyle. (See chapter three on insurance for greater detail.) When dealing with banks or other lending institutions, always know what you want, what you will be assigning as collateral, and how you plan to pay the loan back before you see your banker.

If you are still undecided on how to structure your debt, use the worksheets in this chapter and then ask a loan officer for advice. Remember that banks are primarily in the business of lending money. They write loans so they can afford to pay dividends and create profits for their corporation. Strive to have a positive relationship with your bank, but never work with a bank that bullies you or does not keep your situation in strict confidence. Never lie to your banker—or do anything other than what you specify—since bankers make decisions based on the four Cs of banking: credit, character, collateral, and cash flow. In short, make sure that you take every precaution to safeguard your ability to borrow money.

Even if you have excellent cash flow and feel no pinch in making your monthly budget, go through the debt management and budgetary process. See if there is a way to increase your spendable income or increase your ability to create net worth through proper debt management. Remember, making your money work for you now is a critical concept in building toward retirement.

The following ten rules of debt management are intended to clarify for you how to stay in good graces with your debt.

## Rule One

Put away enough liquid assets to equal six months' budget before you go into debt. This means that if your total monthly expenses (including mortgage, school loans, charity, savings, food, entertainment, utilities—everything) total $8,000, you need to accumulate $48,000 as a security net. Therefore, if you earn $10,000 monthly ($2,000 surplus each month) and want a new car that costs $400 a month, you should have the down payment in savings so as not to dip into your security fund. Feel free to consider CDs and conservative mutual funds as liquid assets when faced with setting up your reserve fund, and it's OK to borrow or use a line of credit. Stock portfolios, on the other hand, should be counted on for half their current value.

## Rule Two

Work to increase your monthly "divine surplus." Depending on the security of your job, a surplus of between 10 percent and 40 percent is good. Self-employed physicians would be wise to save upwards of 25 percent if possible, due to the sometimes unstable nature of the work, while those covered by a long-term contract with a hospital or agency of the government, for instance, can usually get away with a 10 percent surplus.

# Rule Three

Total debt payments should not exceed one-third of your income. No more than 25 percent should go to housing (mortgage or rent), while 10 percent or so is appropriate for auto and other debt installment payments.

# Rule Four

Think balance—life is forever. Debt is not a portent that you're on the road to ruin. Don't be convinced that a debt-free life is an ideal. It does not work that way. Consolidate your home, investment properties, home improvements, and other long-term assets into one big loan with a fixed rate and the minimum required payment. (Quickly go on to rule five.)

# Rule Five

Take full advantage of the fact that home loan interest is deductible. To understand the benefit of restructuring your debt to take advantage of this, review Figure 2.2 (Debt Restructuring—New Physician).

# Rule Six

Never pay down your home interest rate by paying points. Instead, go for a fixed rate, fifteen- to thirty-year mortgage that has no points. The idea is to always allow yourself to refinance when interest rates fall.

# Rule Seven

Aspire to be your own banker by paying cash for cars, boats, etc. When anticipating a large purchase, begin saving to a liquid account so that ample cash is available when the time comes.

# Rule Eight

Maintain control over your credit card use. Like other debt vehicles, credit cards offer wonderful freedom. And quite often there are frequent flyer miles to accrue, charities to benefit, and other perks that accompany credit card use without modifying behavior. Be careful, though; credit card debt can quickly escalate beyond control. Adhere to the following guidelines for help in balanced credit card use: (1) If you can't use credit cards responsibly, cut them up and cancel them; and (2) pay off the balance each month.

## Rule Nine

Keep promises, even at difficult moments when the pressure to spend is strongest. Don't play the irresponsible game of justifying aberrant spending behavior as someone else's fault. If you sign the loan application, accept the credit card, or close the deal with the car dealer, it's your responsibility to live up to the commitment, each and every payment. Occasionally, legitimate problems arise and it is necessary to appeal to your banker for relief. Bankers are prepared to help, so don't wait too long if you get in over your head with debts.

## Rule Ten

Don't wait until you lose your job or have a medical crisis to get your debt/liquidity life in order; do it now! Banks will loan you money when you "don't need it" so to speak, but they too often decline when difficulties arise.

# chapter three

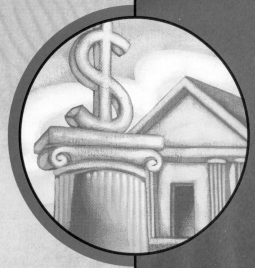

# Carefully Insure Yourself Against Risk and Misfortune

Every physician has witnessed the financial devastation brought on an individual or family due to an accident or illness. Calamities are waiting to happen: the uninsured widow with two children and a spouse dead from an auto accident; a physician's net worth ravaged by malpractice lawsuits; forced retirement due to depression. These are real, everyday affairs that necessitate proper insurance planning. Yes, insurance is a vital part of a well-constructed retirement plan.

Equally important to the risks for which you seek insurance coverage are those you approach with a minimization strategy. Carefully managing your practice, wearing a seat belt, choosing your partners wisely, dealing only with advisors that have clean track records and hefty experience, using off-shore trusts and limited liability corporations, utilizing a privacy policy, and building yourself a sizable nest egg are just some of the noninsurance ways to manage the risks in your life. A book could (and probably should) be written on managing the risks inherent in being a successful physician. The one goal that underscores all of the steps outlined in this book is to be wise about the way you manage the risks of your life. Your financial planner, attorney, and insurance professionals should all be consulted to guide you to a commonsense, reasonably priced insurance risk management program.

Every dollar spent unnecessarily on insurance is a dollar that did not go toward building a retirement nest egg. In my career of working with physicians, I have observed that if more attention had been given to building a lean yet effective insurance portfolio, the average physician could have retired one to two years earlier.

Commisionable whole life insurance, variable life insurance, expensive lump sum or second-to-die policies, or mispriced disability income insurance policies (which flaunt unnecessary bells and whistles) are a few underhanded insurance offerings that are usually excessively expensive and inappropriate. Deductibles, modified premium policies, term insurance, and group policies all can be used to greatly reduce your premium cost, often for similar coverage. Remember, the motivating factor for many insurance agents is commissions. The use of fee-only insurance advisors can not be overemphasized.

On the other hand, otherwise reasonable financial plans have concentrated exclusively on retirement and completely ignored the need for comprehensive and proper risk management. This is a weakness commonly seen amongst plans promoted by some financial planners, be they fee-only or

# Prenuptial Agreements

Prenuptial and postnuptial agreements should be considered by every person contemplating marriage. I realize that this is an incredibly difficult issue for some to discuss before marriage, but the prenuptial can simply be drafted to say in contractual language that a divorce will not ruin your ability to retire with dignity within a reasonable time. It is very reasonable to acknowledge in writing at the beginning of a new marriage that no matter what happens, the wealth accumulated to date is the property of each respective partner. For example, you may wish to have your assets passed on to children or grandchildren, with perhaps a finite amount going to your new spouse in the event of a divorce. This is a sensitive issue and it is best to keep the document simple, straightforward, and reasonable. Seek out an attorney that has experience and sensitivity.

commission-paid planners, lawyers, CPA financial advisors, certified financial planners, or local insurance agents. Too often these plans fail to address the significant risks that can derail even the most solidly constructed financial plan for physicians.

Never insure against a risk that poses only a modest financial effect, such as the need for eyeglasses, incidental dental work, etc. These expenses are not significant enough to disrupt your lifestyle, and you should possess sufficient funds in a liquid account for such eventualities. Insurance should be used only when the potential liability would derail your financial plan. When at all possible, take advantage of the savings offered by deductibles to help reduce the cost of insurance.

# Property and Liability Insurance

Property/liability insurance is vitally important in ensuring that your nest egg and ability to earn and keep a good income are protected. Home owners insurance, auto insurance, and a million dollar plus umbrella liability policy, in addition to life, business, and commercial liability insurance, if needed, all are of great importance to protect you and your business. Having a knowledgeable and seasoned insurance agent representing solid companies should be a top priority. With any plan get a second opinion from an insurance consultant, financial planner, and/or lawyer familiar with insurance.

# Life Insurance

It may seem ironic to discuss life insurance in a retirement planning book, due to the fact that if you're dead all the retirement planning in the world will not matter. However, most of us are concerned about fulfilling the commitments we've made to our spouse, children, business associates, and others, and life insurance will provide at least a financial safety net should you die. Your own ability to retire with security may be jeopardized by the death of a business partner.

Most young physicians have substantial incomes but have not acquired a substantial net worth to assure their family financial security should they die. Figure 3.1 is a Life Insurance Worksheet to help you determine your insurance needs. It is especially important when purchasing life insurance to deal only with a highly rated company. By using the worksheets provided and insurance direct companies (eg, USAA Life Insurance Company, 800 531-8000; Ameritas Life Insurance Corp, 800 745-6665; and AMA Insurance Agency, Inc, 800 458-5736) you can easily control your own life insurance plan.

Figure 3.2 (Sample Term Insurance Rates) shows what top-quality insurance should cost. An attorney or financial advisor can help you designate the ownership and beneficiary designations on your policies.

# Disability Income Insurance

No form of insurance is more important for physicians than disability income insurance from a reputable insurance company. You are a money machine and your primary assets are your skills and your ability to utilize them. If debilitated through sickness or accident, the effect on your financial security would be tremendous; so it is very important to understand exactly what your insurance provides if you're disabled, and even more important to understand how your insurance company defines disabled. A standing joke among insurance agents is that some disability policies are written with such tight restrictions that if you could sell pencils on a street corner, you would not be considered disabled.

On the other end of contract provisions for a disability policy is one that covers you for your specialty. These companies will pay full benefits if you are unable to practice your specialty, even if you are able to practice another area of medicine.

**Figure 3.1**

# Life Insurance Worksheet

## Step 1

List below who would suffer financially if you died (eg, spouse, children, parents, business partners, charity, friends, siblings).

**Name**          **Type of loss (eg, income, debt payback, family care)**

_____

_____

_____

_____

## Step 2

Assign a specific amount of economic support for the above-listed people.

Monthly income to _____ of $ _____

Monthly income to _____ of $ _____

Pay off debts of $_____ for _____

Cash resource of $_____ for _____

Special cash to _____ of $ _____ lump sum.

## Step 3

Total monthly income desired at $_____ ÷ 0.005 = $_____

Total cash needed to pay off debts and
mortgages, for cash reserves, and special cash =    $_____

Total assets needed to provide for above =    $_____
(A 6% interest rate is used so that excess earnings
can go to help offset inflation.)

Total assets needed (from above) =    $_____

Less liquid assets you own and assets that
could be made liquid =    $_____

**Total insurance death benefit you need =**    $_____

## Figure 3.2

# Sample Term Insurance Rates

$1 million of term coverage at nonsmoker-preferred rates

| | Male | | | | | | Age | | Female | | | | |
|---|---|---|---|---|---|---|---|---|---|---|---|---|---|
| ART* | 5 Years | 10 Years | 15 Years | 20 Years | 30 Years | | | ART* | 5 Years | 10 Years | 15 Years | 20 Years | 30 Years |
| $ 630 | $ 480 | $ 340 | $ 570 | $ 630 | $ 930 | | 25 | $ 470 | $ 390 | $ 320 | $ 460 | $ 540 | $ 710 |
| 630 | 480 | 350 | 580 | 640 | 970 | | 30 | 490 | 390 | 330 | 480 | 550 | 750 |
| 670 | 480 | 350 | 590 | 640 | 1,090 | | 35 | 510 | 390 | 330 | 490 | 550 | 830 |
| 790 | 690 | 510 | 870 | 920 | 1,560 | | 40 | 580 | 560 | 380 | 690 | 710 | 1,120 |
| 1,010 | 1,010 | 830 | 1,290 | 1,420 | 2,390 | | 45 | 720 | 780 | 530 | 970 | 1,020 | 1,620 |
| 1,290 | 1,530 | 1,290 | 2,020 | 2,120 | 3,900 | | 50 | 910 | 1,090 | 820 | 1,410 | 1,480 | 2,680 |
| 1,770 | 2,290 | 2,040 | 3,170 | 3,400 | N/A | | 55 | 1,130 | 1,550 | 1,310 | 2,040 | 2,300 | N/A |
| 5,300 | $6,480 | 5,870 | 8,270 | N/A | N/A | | 65 | 2,970 | 3,650 | 3,290 | 4,820 | N/A | N/A |

* ART = Guaranteed annually renewable and convertible term premium.

Rates supplied by Ameritas Life Insurance Corp, 800 745-6665; USAA Life Insurance Company, 800 531-8000); and Schwab Insurance Direct, 800 838-0650.

# Be Prepared for Anything

Health care is a dynamic, rapidly changing, billion dollar industry with literally thousands of highly trained professionals working to improve delivery efficacy and cost-effectiveness. Physicians act as the hub of the many-spoked wheel of medicine—working with patients, employers, the scientific world, and virtually everyone else. Along with being breathlessly paced, this dubious position also makes them the most susceptible to change. As employees, they may be laid off just like any factory worker, or forced out of work because at midcareer they have finally learned to say an adamant *no* to teaching classes on Saturday mornings, mentoring new residents, sitting on the ethics committee, being part of a finance review board, or anything else that takes time away from family and friends. Over the course of a career, more and more duties and responsibilities are added until the wheel finally breaks down and a once energetic physician finds him- or herself burned out, uninspired, tired, and frustrated. The few who have learned to say no and to make time to enjoy Saturday mornings with the family, Friday nights watching a daughter play basketball, or Wednesdays learning Spanish are those labeled uncooperative,

lazy, and not a team player, and are consequently the first to go when the practice buyout happens.

When you work for somebody else or simply confront the possibility that you could lose your license to an innocent mistake, you must prepare financially and emotionally *to lose your job.* Such a predicament requires that you have great liquidity and your budget under control.

Also, understand that health care delivery is a competitive job market. One of the ways you can prepare for eventual mishaps is to treat current employees and employers with respect (even if they don't deserve it) so that if you need to seek another job, at least your coworkers will say you were a good physician who got along with everybody. Everyone you work with might be asked to give you a reference.

Your contract should be designed to protect you from involuntary or voluntary separation. You might suggest that for each year you have worked for your employer, you get a month's severance should there be a separation. That way, if after six years your employer is bought out and your services become redundant, you will receive six months' salary as you search for a new job.

Figure 3.3 (Disability Income Insurance Worksheet) may be utilized to help you decide how much disability income insurance you will need to support your lifestyle (unless you have sufficient personal assets to negate the need for disability insurance). It will also help you decide what elimination period you should have on your policy. An elimination period is the number of days you must wait before you receive a benefit from your policy. Generally it runs from a thirty-day wait (substantially more expensive) to a two-year wait.

Key contract provisions you should have in your policy are outlined in Figure 3.4 (Key Contract Provisions). In addition to the provisions listed, another way to structure your policy is as a graded or step premium policy, which keeps your premiums low for a few years, then gradually increases them until the premium levels off after a certain period. Graded premium or guaranteed annual renewable policies are especially helpful for the younger physician who needs a substantial amount of quality protection but has a limited budget. These policies are an excellent buy; however, they are usually available only to physicians under the age of fifty.

A policy with a future increase option benefit allows you to purchase more disability income insurance regardless of your future health; so if you suddenly develop diabetes or a back problem after purchasing your policy, you can increase policy benefits without any riders or waivers on your health problems. This is a good choice for physicians who foresee having substantial salary increases and plan on purchasing additional disability insurance in the future.

Expect to pay a healthy premium for the best disability coverage. It is far better to have a $2,000/month policy with very favorable contract provisions than to have a policy that will pay you $4,000 a month but has limitations and loopholes.

**Figure 3.3**

# Disability Income Insurance Worksheet

A. Amount of monthly income you need to support your lifestyle                 $_____
   (debt payments, utilities, food, entertainment, education, etc)

B. Current investments that could be quickly converted to cash                 $_____

   Divided by monthly income needed                                           ÷ $_____

   Equals number of months personal funds will support you                    = _____

C. Income expected should you become disabled:

   1st month $_____        2nd month $_____        3rd month $_____

## Elimination Period Calculation

Number of months receivables will support you                                  _____

Plus number of months liquid investments will support you                    + _____

Equals the elimination period in months                                      = _____

Income needed to support your lifestyle                                        $_____

Subtract income from assets not figured in liquidity elimination
period analysis, such as pension plan assets, IRA, income
partnerships, etc; multiply the value of these assets by .005                 = $_____
(for example, $1,000,000 x .005 = $5,000 monthly)

**Amount of income needed from disability income insurance**                   $_____

*Note:* Benefit period should always be at least to age 65 for sickness or accident, and usually lifetime for both
         sickness and accident.

## Figure 3.4

# Key Contract Provisions

| Important Contract Provision | Benefit and Importance of Provision |
|---|---|
| 1. Payment at age 65 or lifetime benefit, if possible | Pays you at least to age 65 to provide long-term security. |
| 2. Favorable definition of disability, regarding either (a) "Your Occupation" or (b) "With Residual." | **"Your Occupation"** definition protects your ability to earn a living doing what you do now. This policy will pay you even if you work in another profession.<br><br>**"With Residual"** benefit provides a benefit tied to either earnings lost or percent of time spent at occupation lost due to disability. A benefit based on earnings lost is far superior to time lost and should always be purchased. In fact, an "earnings lost" residual policy is better than a "your occupation" policy. Some policies pay full benefits even if you earn up to 49% of your predisability pay. |
| 3. Cost of living/inflation protection benefit | Postdisability benefits can increase with inflation, ie, price increases. Minimum increase you should purchase is 3% a year up to three times policy benefit (current benefit of $4,000 monthly could raise to $12,000 monthly maximum). Some policies increase benefits regardless of inflation rate. |
| 4. Noncancelable/guaranteed renewable coverage | Policy cannot be changed by anyone except you. Premiums are guaranteed not to increase above level stated in policy. |
| 5. Subsequent disability reoccurrence provision | Waives a new elimination period if, following a disability, you become disabled again from the same or another cause. |
| 6. Earnings definition should include pension contributions and all bonuses | Helps ensure you will get residual benefit. |
| 7. Preexisting conditions covered if listed on policy application | Some policies cover only sickness or accidents first "manifest" while policy is in force; eg, supposing you had back problems in high school; company could deny claim based on injury prior to buying policy. |

*Note:* Your disability income insurance policy is the most important insurance you can own. Make sure your policy fits your needs completely and has no loopholes.

# Offshore Trusts

If your personal assets, not including your retirement plan and home, total $1 million dollars or more, you should consider an offshore asset protection trust (APT). While controversial and often used for other reasons, an APT can prevent your assets from becoming a litigation target.

To illustrate just how dramatic the results of an APT can be, consider the case of a physician who fell prey several years ago to negative publicity that consequently spawned a spate of lawsuits. As reported in the financial press, he fought them all. When he tired of the traditional legal battle and associated costs, he decided to switch tactics by setting up an APT. Although his attorneys were careful to leave him with enough assets to cover potential damage awards, his "pot of gold" in the form of bank accounts, stocks, and bonds was no longer accessible to his conniving suitors. In the end he settled all fifteen cases (for which he was uninsured) for less than $18,000. Moreover, his savings could have been much more dramatic if he had set up an APT before the legal travails.

Economics drive the legal system, and deep pockets are the primary motivation of any lawsuit. Therein lies the most attractive benefit of an APT: financial prophylaxis. Once you recognize that incorporation and liability insurance aren't impenetrable, and that the courts are continually defining new rights for plaintiffs at the expense of those with the gold, it's easy to appreciate the benefits of an APT.

The goal of preserving, protecting, and arranging for the ultimate distribution of assets to your designated beneficiaries is accomplished when an APT is set up in conjunction with a family limited partnership (FLP). The result is very nearly an impenetrable wall against future creditors, which is not the case with an FLP alone. By establishing an FLP, you own the partnership interest rather than the assets transferred. When you add an APT, you reduce the size of your estate available to creditors, while still retaining control.

An APT simply sets up a trust in countries that do not recognize the legal jurisdiction of US courts in civil disputes. They usually operate within the same legal principles and offer the same protections as some trusts used in the United States. Notably different is the fact that with an APT you can control the assets, provided you select the right jurisdiction. Should they wish to, creditors are required to pursue your assets under the jurisdiction of the foreign country.

Asset protection planning is a "what if" endeavor to protect your assets in advance of some financial calamity. What if you were sued for professional negligence and your personal assets were exposed because of limited malpractice insurance coverage, an insurer's insolvency, or punitive damages (which generally are not covered)? A host of other tort claims may arise from business, personal, or financial affairs: Your dog bites the mail carrier. Something happens in your swimming pool or on your trampoline. The applicable legal doctrine is fraudulent conveyance, meaning you can't hide assets after the fact.

It is inaccurate to view APTs as tax shelters because they are tax neutral. They have no particular income, gift, or estate tax advantage other than the same found in inter vivos or testamentary trusts. So if your interest in an APT is for tax evasion purposes, forget it.

*continued on next page*

## Offshore Trusts continued

Nor is an APT a means to defraud creditors. If an APT is set up for an individual desiring protection—when they have no pending or threatened claims or reason to believe that a legal problem will develop— no argument that the APT was intended to defraud creditors will prevail. On the other hand, if an APT was created when an individual was on the brink of bankruptcy, fraudulent conveyance laws would come into effect. The conveyance laws look at the intent of the transferor at the time of the transfer of assets to an APT.

Nor is an APT appropriate for hiding assets. Although it offers confidentiality, full disclosure is necessary on your tax return.

For some physicians, ironclad security is the ultimate appeal of an APT. They value knowing that no matter what happens, no one can get to their home or nonretirement plan assets. (Homes and retirement plans are protected from liability claims in most states.)

When choosing a site to establish an APT, realize that not all foreign countries offer the same benefits. Choose one that has a long legal history based on English common law. Political stability is also critical, as is thorough asset protection–style trust law.

Although most offshore trust companies will walk you through the process, retaining an attorney is still necessary. Legal fees of up to $15,000 can be expected, as well as some travel costs. Annual maintenance fees run about $2,000 per year.

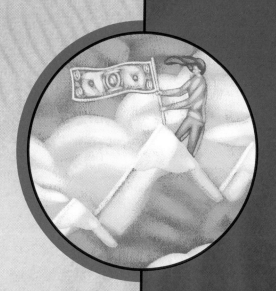

# chapter four

# Control Taxes

Taxes are the biggest personal budget item for physicians. Yet through the wise use of tax-qualified retirement plans and other tax savings strategies, physicians can add efficiency to their present tax situation to enhance their bid for retirement happiness. In earlier chapters we discussed using tax-deductible interest strategies to reduce the after-tax cost of managing your debt. The use of business forms such as limited liability corporations for risk management can also be helpful in tax planning. This chapter will go a long way in helping you understand the important role tax savings and planning play as part of a comprehensive retirement plan.

The number one retirement priority for every physician should be to fund—to the maximum—a tax-favored retirement plan. The use of tax-favored retirement plans is the core strategy of this book; its importance cannot be overemphasized. Tax-qualified retirement plans have three distinct tax benefits: (1) contributions are currently tax-deductible; (2) earnings on plan assets grow tax-free; and (3) withdrawals are flexible at retirement. Figure 4.1 (Why Use Qualified Retirement Plans) illustrates the advantages of tax-qualified retirement plans.

Not so wonderful is the fact that tax-qualified retirement plans have annual contribution limits (see Figure 6.1, Comparison of Plans for Retirement, for a review of contribution limits for different plans). Also, if you miss funding your retirement plan one year (except in rare cases), you can never make up for that lost year's deposit. These stipulations reinforce the importance of funding your retirement plan to the max every year. Even first-year residents should consider funding, at least, Roth IRAs due to their significant benefits.

Figure 4.1 shows that $1,000 placed in a tax-deductible plan will save you $400 if you are in a 40 percent tax bracket, and that your net worth will grow by the whole $1,000. Similarly, if you place the maximum $30,000 into a money purchase retirement plan, Uncle Sam will, in theory, write out a contribution check to you equal to your tax bracket. For example, a 40 percent tax bracket would earn a check of $12,000. If you funded your plan at $30,000 a year for twenty-five years with a 6 percent return, Uncle Sam's contribution alone would be worth nearly $700,000.

Tax-qualified retirement plans grow tax-deferred. Tax-deferred means that the taxes on your deductible deposit and its growth are not levied until you draw on your account. Annuities issued by insurance companies also grow tax-free, as do cash value life insurance policies. Although blessed with tax benefits, insurance annuities and life insurance policies are usually not effective capital accumulators due to a cost structure that ravages any tax

**Figure 4.1**

# Why Use Qualified Retirement Plans

## Contributions are currently tax-deductible

**Example:**  $1,000.00  placed in plan
– 400.00  tax saved at 40% tax bracket
$  600.00  net cost to build net worth by $1,000.00

## Earnings on plan assets grow tax-free

**Example:**  $1,000.00  monthly at 6% not taxed  = $  462,000 in 20 years
= $1,004,000 in 30 years

$  600.00  monthly at 6% less 40% tax = 3.6% net return
= $350,000 in 20 years
= $646,640 in 30 years

## Lots of money in retirement plan = Lots of income at retirement

**Example:**  $1,000.00  monthly at 6%  = $  462,000 in 20 years = $2,310/month
at 6%
$1,004,000 in 30 years = $5,020/month
at 6%

$  600.00  monthly at 6%  = 3.6% net return
$  350,000 in 20 years = $1,750/month
at 6%
$  646,640 in 30 years = $3,233/month
at 6%

*Note:* This illustration is oversimplified; however, it accurately highlights the tax benefits of a retirement plan, not to mention the liability protection. Also, note that the monthly income difference is nearly $1,800 in the 30-year example.

# Use It or Lose It

Every resident should strive to fund Roth IRAs and, if possible, Tax Sheltered 403(b) plans (TSAs) with their meager resident salaries, *even if it means your student loans will be larger.* Why? Taxes and the fact that the IRS limits how much you can contribute each year to these very tax beneficial retirement plans.

Let's say you're a twenty-six-year-old first-year resident making $22,000 a year and you fund a non-tax-deductible Roth during a four-year residency at $2,000 each year ($166/monthly). That $8,000 will grow completely tax-free until your age is 59½, at which time you will have $54,000 if it grows at 6 percent, which is a reasonable, after-inflation net rate. For gains at a 10 percent return, you will have $177,000 for your $8,000 sacrifice and, since it's a Roth, you can take your money out *completely tax-free* anytime you want after reaching age 59½.

While funding a TSA is not as valuable as contributing to a Roth IRA, it's still a compelling strategy if you can afford it. TSA 403(b) plans are salary reduction plans you set up with your university; these plans allow you to put up to 20 percent of your assets into no-load mutual funds or annuities. The contributions are before-tax and are taken right out of your paycheck before you see the money. The account grows tax-deferred, so you don't pay taxes on it until you take it out at retirement.

Continuing with our twenty-six-year-old resident example, if she puts 20 percent of her $22,000 into the TSA, she will be saving an additional $4,400 annually, or $367 monthly, for her four-year residency. At the end of her residency, she will have saved $17,600, which will be worth $19,835 at 6 percent after four years. Growing at 6 percent, it will be worth $118,863 by the time she reaches age sixty; figured "for grins" at 10 percent, it would be $390,000. Wow! $17,600 sure does grow over time!

---

Got kids or grandchildren? The above strategy is great and works well for anyone. If you have extra assets and are in the gifting mood, help them out by gifting to them a Roth IRA or the ability to fund the TSA. It's worth over ten times more to them now than at their retirement.

---

benefits. Real estate, growth common stocks, gold, silver, collectibles, antiques, and other assets purchased for investment that grow without throwing off much income (whose return comes from growth in value) also have tax-deferred characteristics.

Even while tax-qualified retirement plans are tax-deductible and tax-deferred, eventually (except Roth IRAs, which have tax-free withdrawals at retirement) you will have to pay the tax man. But, as Figure 4.2 (Quantifying the Retirement Plan) shows, you are still way ahead using them as the cornerstone of your retirement plan. For example, if you are saving $2,000 monthly toward retirement in a qualified retirement plan, in thirty years (assuming 6 percent interest) you will have $2 million, which

# Figure 4.2

# Quantifying the Retirement Plan

Pension or IRA/TSA Breakeven Holding Periods Average Annual Yield to Withdrawal (including 10% penalty for nonsystematic withdrawal before age 59½)*

| Constant Marginal Tax Rate | Average Return per Period | | | | | | | | | | | |
|---|---|---|---|---|---|---|---|---|---|---|---|---|
| | 6% | 7% | 8% | 9% | 10% | 11% | 12% | 13% | 14% | 15% | 16% | 17% |
| 10% | 19.63 | 16.83 | 14.72 | 13.09 | 11.78 | 10.71 | 9.82 | 9.06 | 8.41 | 7.85 | 7.36 | 6.93 |
| 15 | 13.91 | 11.92 | 10.43 | 9.27 | 8.34 | 7.59 | 6.95 | 6.42 | 5.96 | 5.56 | 5.22 | 4.91 |
| 20 | 11.13 | 9.54 | 8.35 | 7.42 | 6.68 | 6.07 | 5.56 | 5.14 | 4.77 | 4.45 | 4.17 | 3.93 |
| 25 | 9.54 | 8.18 | 7.16 | 6.36 | 5.72 | 5.20 | 4.77 | 4.40 | 4.09 | 3.82 | 3.58 | 3.37 |
| 30 | 8.56 | 7.34 | 6.42 | 5.71 | 5.14 | 4.67 | 4.28 | 3.95 | 3.67 | 3.43 | 3.21 | 3.02 |
| 35 | 7.0 | 6.82 | 5.97 | 5.30 | 4.77 | 4.34 | 3.98 | 3.67 | 3.41 | 3.18 | 2.98 | 2.81 |
| 40 | 7.60 | 6.51 | 5.70 | 5.06 | 4.56 | 4.14 | 3.80 | 3.51 | 3.26 | 3.04 | 2.85 | 2.68 |
| 45 | 7.43 | 6.37 | 5.57 | 4.95 | 4.46 | 4.05 | 3.72 | 3.43 | 3.19 | 2.97 | 2.79 | 2.62 |
| 50 | 7.44 | 6.38 | 5.58 | 4.69 | 4.46 | 4.06 | 3.72 | 3.43 | 3.19 | 2.98 | 2.79 | 2.63 |

* Rates are continuously compounded for both taxes and average annual yield. Rates not continuously compounded can be substituted for a rough idea of the breakeven point. Example: If you are in a 40% tax bracket and you earn 8% on your tax-qualified retirement plan, in a little over 5 1/2 years, you will be at "breakeven." This means that even if you cashed in your IRA and paid a 10% penalty plus current income tax on your withdrawal, you would be ahead if you did it after 5.7 years (over not having had an IRA, TSA, or pension plan).

Planning tips: Worried about educating the kids? This chart shows how even after all tax consequences of an early withdrawal, it still usually makes sense to max out on retirement plans. Concerned you don't have enough "liquidity funds," so are forgoing your retirement plan contribution? Take the risk and fund your plan is usually the best after-analysis.

would give you $10,000 monthly income, before taxes. If your $2,000 monthly savings is after-tax (in the 40 percent tax bracket), your net savings is $1,200 monthly, which in thirty years will be worth $1,293,000 and will provide you with an income of only $6,465 monthly, before taxes. As you can see, over time a tax-qualified retirement plan can increase the efficiency of your savings plan by 50 percent or more depending on your rate of return, tax bracket, and time frame.

# Using Professionals

A good retirement plan advisor can be a tremendous ally in helping you find the best tax-qualified plan(s). It is equally important to have your tax return completed by a competent tax preparer who is well trained and familiar with the unique needs of physicians. Any tax strategies that you consider should be reviewed by your tax advisor before they are implemented. Frequently, salespeople will call you with tax schemes promising surefire benefits that seem to be consistent with current tax law. But no matter how logical they sound, you should first have a trusted advisor review such strategies. If you choose to take an aggressive tax stance, make sure that you have a letter from a large tax-oriented law firm or Big Five accounting firm stating that the strategy is appropriate, honest, and consistent with the law, and that it fits your tax situation. This should be done before you go to the hassle and expense of implementing any questionable strategy.

# A Word on Mutual Funds Taxes

In magazines like *Barron's, Money,* and *Fortune,* the mutual fund industry shamelessly touts the performance of top mutual fund managers. No one, on the other hand, seems to talk about their after-tax investment performance. If you're looking for a dark secret of the industry, check out why many funds are not forthcoming about this fact.

With IRAs, 401ks, and tax-exempt retirement plans, it doesn't make any difference what the capital gains consequences are in a mutual fund. However, in your taxable accounts—where you are paying on all the dividends and capital gains generated—the after-tax cost can be incredibly painful.

Since most physicians are in the highest tax brackets, understanding the after-tax return on your portfolio is of paramount concern. The most important thing to understand is that when you buy a mutual fund, you inherit the capital gains that are already embedded in the mutual fund portfolio.

If you bought the portfolio on January 1 with a price tag of $20 a share, and on January 2 it sells off a portion of investments and declares a capital gain of $5 a share, you have to pay taxes on that $5 even though you did not own the fund when those gains were made. Therefore, when you purchase mutual funds for your taxable accounts, make sure that:

1. You purchase portfolios that don't have a lot of embedded capital gains.

2. The turnover of the portfolio is small.

3. You accept that you have significant capital gains and trust the management will outperform the tax consequences.

If your portfolio is $250,000 or more, you should not use funds. Instead, consider an individually managed portfolio guided by a competent fee-only professional.

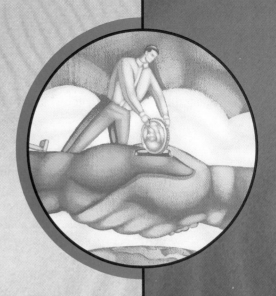

# chapter five

# Save

Noncompliant patients, 5 AM surgeries, on-call weekends, and missed dinners all can get old quickly and make you think about retiring sooner rather than later. While most physicians find their work fulfilling, much like eating excess ice cream, too much work can make you sick.

In preparing for a successful retirement, the key to flourishing on the wealth you have created is saving an appropriate amount of money. In most cases, this requires the development of systems and processes that facilitate your desire to set aside part of your income for retirement. Nearly every physician can retire with ease. The goal of a well-constructed retirement plan is to add efficiency so that you can retire earlier, have more spendable income now, and live a balanced life.

There are many uncomplicated, painless strategies you can utilize to save money that will add up to a hefty nest egg. Take a look at Figure 5.1 (When Saving for Retirement, Simple Things Add Up). Retirement success requires that you concentrate on building net worth in a wise and carefully planned methodology. In fact, all the chapters in this book offer ways that you can reduce your outgo for taxes, insurance, etc, so that you can save more toward building net worth.

# Retire in Ten Years

If you are willing to sacrifice and stay disciplined, retiring in ten years is well within your reach, even if you are a physician fresh out of residency. Figure 5.2 (Retire in Ten Years) tells you exactly what you need to save in order to pull off an accelerated retirement schedule.

Of course, saving is the penultimate key to retiring early. Naturally, the job is greatly eased by starting as soon as possible and saving as much as possible. Remember to take these steps:

- Control taxes in order to be more efficient.
- Closely monitor your budget and manage debts as illustrated and outlined in chapters one and two.
- Make sure your insurance program is lean, mean, and appropriate.
- Invest wisely (how to do so is covered in later chapters).

Contrary to popular belief, tax-sheltered retirement plans do not require you to wait until age 60 to draw on them. The IRS merely requires that if you

# Sell Your Practice

Added income for retirement can come from the sale of or interest in your practice. But what is it worth—or more importantly, what will your practice be worth at retirement? The textbook answer would be whatever a willing buyer would pay and what you would be willing to sell it for. History, however, has given us some precedents that deserve your attention.

A good solo practice is worth 40 percent of receipts. If the practice is bringing in $300,000 in revenues, then it is worth somewhere in the vicinity of $120,000. But a practice with $300,000 in revenues is worth a lot more (percentage wise) than a practice that brings in only $80,000. Similarly, a practice earning $500,000 may be worth up to 70 percent of receipts, depending on the practice and the number of patients available for conversion to capitation. As with most generalizations, there are many caveats involved in these numbers.

So what is your practice worth as part of your retirement plan? *Nothing!* Nothing except the estimate of hard value at retirement. You'll notice throughout this book that this is the only place we mention the value of your practice, only to say that it's worth nothing.

It is important that you not count on your practice being worth much when planning, but as you get nearer to retirement you can begin to account for its value and add it to your plan. It is effective to view the value of your practice in terms of how many months or years it will buy you in retirement. If you anticipate selling it for $120,000, and that happens to be your yearly budget in retirement, you can count on it for one year.

start drawing on your retirement plan before age 59½, you must draw consistent amounts annually until age 59½, or five years, whichever is longer. For example, if you're able to accumulate $1 million in your retirement plan by age 45 due to great investment returns and good savings habits, you could draw $5,000 monthly from the account for your life, but you could not reduce that amount before age 59½ without a tax penalty. However, if you go back to work and decide you don't need the $5,000 a month, most likely you would have to either receive it or pay a 10 percent tax penalty on all withdrawals made.

# Save 10 Percent

As a rule of thumb, try to save at least 10 percent of your income each year during your career. During a career that lasts thirty-five years, saving 10 percent and earning 6 percent interest (a worthy

**The average fee-only financial advisor serving physicians found that . . .**
Their average client saves $25,000 to $30,000 in tax-qualified retirement plans and $5,000 to $50,000 outside of plans yearly, with older physicians saving significantly more than younger physicians.

**Figure 5.1**

# When Saving for Retirement, Simple Things Add Up

1. Say no to any commissionable, cash value life insurance—age 35 male, $1 million policy. Buy no-commission term instead. Approximate five-year savings at $10,000* – Value at age 60 =    $   33,000

2. Say yes to placing savings on life insurance into a tax-qualified plan. Add at age 60 =    $   27,000

3. Say yes to using group policies, annual renewable, and step rate disability policies, in addition to decreasing policies as needs change and net worth grows. Estimated savings at $1,000/year =    $   57,000

4. Say yes to using frequent flyer credit cards. Estimate use at $35,000/year = One round-trip ticket to Hawaii at $950 – $50 credit card fee = $900 per year =    $   52,000

5. Use fee-only investment advisors who invest at low commissions with reasonable fees and/or use no load, low-fee mutual funds like Vanguard and TIAA/CREF. Estimate 1% additional returns on $30,000 annual savings =    $  244,000

6. Use tax-qualified retirement plans instead of after-tax savings ($30,000/year deposit to retirement plan) =    $  693,000

7. Invest two-thirds of your 6 months' liquidity account in short-term bond mutual fund, short-term municipal bonds instead of money market only, to earn an additional 1% on $60,000 =    $   34,000

8. Live your life with long-term orientation—relax and "smell the roses" all through your career. Make "I worked if I wanted, how I wanted, when I wanted, and where I wanted" your work motto. Enjoy your life so much you "retire" 10 years later. Estimate value at age 70 =    $1,838,000

* Assumes 6% return on savings, 40% tax bracket, age 35 physician, and retirement at age 60.

---

**Figure 5.2**

# Retire in Ten Years

Your current investment portfolio value as a percent of your current annual income

Percent of income you need to save, assuming it earns 6%, to have 50% of your income replaced by drawing on your portfolio at 6% (to retire in . . .)

| Percent | 10 Years | 15 Years | 20 Years |
|---------|----------|----------|----------|
| 0       | 60       | 34       | 21       |
| 100     | 54       | 30       | 17       |
| 200     | 47       | 25       | 13       |
| 300     | 41       | 19       | 9        |
| 400     | 34       | 14       | 5        |
| 500     | 23       | 9        | 0        |

*Example:* A physician earning $100,000 a year who had $200,000 in investments would need to save 47% of his or her earnings, or $47,000 annually, to have $1 million in 10 years. $1 million at 6% would give an income of approximately $60,000. I use 6% because you need to have excess income and growth in your portfolio to offset inflation. Due to taxes, the best place to save usually is in a tax-deductible pension profit-sharing plan, 401k, TSA, IRA, etc. How do you retire early? Save what you can, invest wisely, and be patient.

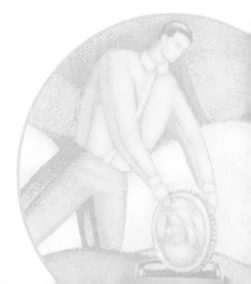

goal is to earn 6 percent more than inflation so that you will retire success-fully with income in real dollars of today) will give you 70 percent of your salary at retirement. With the judicious use of tax-sheltered retirement plans, you could save 16 percent of your income which, after taxes, only affects your budget by 10 percent. After a thirty-five-year career, you would have 110 percent of your preretirement income. If you save 16 percent, the 10 percent effect on your budget after only thirty years will allow you 80 percent of your preretirement income. Chapter one discusses how much retirement income is necessary to support the lifestyle you desire. Because of the many subjective variables, there is no good rule of thumb about how much retirement income is sufficient as a percentage of preretirement income. Everybody is different. Some physicians will find they spend more in retirement than they did before retirement, and others will find just the opposite.

Chapter one helped you come up with the lump sum amount you'll need to retire, based on your goals and needs. By now you might have a good idea of what you can save on a monthly basis, and you also might have figured out your investment risk tolerance (risk tolerance is discussed in chapter seven). You are now prepared to use the Retirement Reality Worksheet (Figure 5.3), which will explain "how much to get how much."

**Figure 5.3**

# Retirement Reality Worksheet

## Retirement Reality

1. Lump sum needed (from chapter one)  $_____

2. How much you have saved so far for retirement  $_____
   (see step 1, below)

3. Estimate how much you can save annually for retirement  $_____

4. In how many years do you wish to retire?  _____

## Reality Test

**Step 1:** Value of lump sum $_____ ×* _____ =  $_____
(*Factor from lump sum "future value factors" as
shown in Figure 5.4)

**Step 2:** Value of annual savings $_____ ×* _____ =  $_____
(*Factor from future value of $1 per year as shown
in Figure 5.5)

**Step 3:** Add sum of steps 1 and 2 =  $_____

How close is this sum to the lump sum needed figure from step 1 above?
If it is more, you will be able to retire earlier if you wish; if it is less, you know the answer.

## Figure 5.4

# Future Value Factors for Lump Sum of $1

| Years | 3% | 4% | 5% | 6% | 7% | 8% | 9% | 10% |
|---|---|---|---|---|---|---|---|---|
| 1 | 1.0300 | 1.0400 | 1.0500 | 1.0600 | 1.0700 | 1.0800 | 1.0900 | 1.1000 |
| 2 | 1.0609 | 1.0816 | 1.1025 | 1.1236 | 1.1449 | 1.1664 | 1.1881 | 1.2100 |
| 3 | 1.0927 | 1.1249 | 1.1576 | 1.1910 | 1.2250 | 1.2597 | 1.2950 | 1.3310 |
| 4 | 1.1255 | 1.1699 | 1.2155 | 1.2625 | 1.3108 | 1.3605 | 1.4116 | 1.4641 |
| 5 | 1.1593 | 1.2167 | 1.2763 | 1.3382 | 1.4026 | 1.4693 | 1.5386 | 1.6105 |
| 6 | 1.1941 | 1.2653 | 1.3401 | 1.4185 | 1.5007 | 1.5869 | 1.6771 | 1.7716 |
| 7 | 1.2299 | 1.3159 | 1.4071 | 1.5036 | 1.6058 | 1.7138 | 1.8280 | 1.9487 |
| 8 | 1.2668 | 1.3686 | 1.4775 | 1.5938 | 1.7182 | 1.8509 | 1.9926 | 2.1436 |
| 9 | 1.3048 | 1.4233 | 1.5513 | 1.6895 | 1.8385 | 1.9990 | 2.1719 | 2.3579 |
| 10 | 1.3439 | 1.4802 | 1.6289 | 1.7908 | 1.9672 | 2.1589 | 2.3674 | 2.5937 |
| 11 | 1.3842 | 1.5395 | 1.7103 | 1.8983 | 2.1049 | 2.3316 | 2.5804 | 2.8531 |
| 12 | 1.4258 | 1.6010 | 1.7959 | 2.0122 | 2.2522 | 2.5182 | 2.8127 | 3.1384 |
| 13 | 1.4685 | 1.6651 | 1.8856 | 2.1329 | 2.4098 | 2.7196 | 3.0658 | 3.4523 |
| 14 | 1.5126 | 1.7317 | 1.9799 | 2.2609 | 2.5785 | 2.9372 | 3.3417 | 3.7975 |
| 15 | 1.5580 | 1.8009 | 2.0789 | 2.3966 | 2.7590 | 3.1722 | 3.6425 | 4.1772 |
| 16 | 1.6047 | 1.8730 | 2.1829 | 2.5404 | 2.9522 | 3.4259 | 3.9703 | 4.5950 |
| 17 | 1.6528 | 1.9479 | 2.2920 | 2.6928 | 3.1588 | 3.7000 | 4.3276 | 5.0545 |
| 18 | 1.7024 | 2.0258 | 2.4066 | 2.8543 | 3.3799 | 3.9960 | 4.7171 | 5.5599 |
| 19 | 1.7535 | 2.1068 | 2.5270 | 3.0256 | 3.6165 | 4.3157 | 5.1417 | 6.1159 |
| 20 | 1.8061 | 2.1911 | 2.6533 | 3.2071 | 3.8697 | 4.6610 | 5.6044 | 6.7275 |
| 21 | 1.8603 | 2.2788 | 2.7860 | 3.3996 | 4.1406 | 5.0338 | 6.1088 | 7.4003 |
| 22 | 1.9161 | 2.3699 | 2.9253 | 3.6035 | 4.4304 | 5.4365 | 6.6586 | 8.1403 |
| 23 | 1.9736 | 2.4647 | 3.0715 | 3.8197 | 4.7405 | 5.8715 | 7.2579 | 8.9543 |
| 24 | 2.0328 | 2.5633 | 3.2251 | 4.0489 | 5.0724 | 6.3412 | 7.9111 | 9.8497 |
| 25 | 2.0938 | 2.6658 | 3.3864 | 4.2919 | 5.4274 | 6.8485 | 8.6231 | 10.8347 |
| 26 | 2.1566 | 2.7725 | 3.5557 | 4.5494 | 5.8074 | 7.3964 | 9.3992 | 11.9182 |

**Figure 5.4** *continued*

| Years | 3% | 4% | 5% | 6% | 7% | 8% | 9% | 10% |
|-------|------|------|------|------|------|------|------|------|
| 27 | 2.2213 | 2.8834 | 3.7335 | 4.8223 | 6.2139 | 7.9881 | 10.2451 | 13.1100 |
| 28 | 2.2879 | 2.9987 | 3.9201 | 5.1117 | 6.6488 | 8.6271 | 11.1671 | 14.4210 |
| 29 | 2.3566 | 3.1187 | 4.1161 | 5.4184 | 7.1143 | 9.3173 | 12.1722 | 15.8631 |
| 30 | 2.4273 | 3.2434 | 4.3219 | 5.7435 | 7.6123 | 10.0627 | 13.2677 | 17.4494 |
| 31 | 2.5001 | 3.3731 | 4.5380 | 6.0881 | 8.1451 | 10.8677 | 14.4618 | 19.1943 |
| 32 | 2.5751 | 3.5081 | 4.7649 | 6.4534 | 8.7153 | 11.7371 | 15.7633 | 21.1138 |
| 33 | 2.6523 | 3.6484 | 5.0032 | 6.8406 | 9.3253 | 12.6761 | 17.1820 | 23.2252 |
| 34 | 2.7319 | 3.7943 | 5.2533 | 7.2510 | 9.9781 | 13.6901 | 18.7284 | 25.5477 |
| 35 | 2.8139 | 3.9461 | 5.5160 | 7.6861 | 10.6766 | 14.7853 | 20.4140 | 28.1024 |
| 36 | 2.8983 | 4.1039 | 5.7918 | 8.1473 | 11.4239 | 15.9682 | 22.2512 | 30.9128 |
| 37 | 2.9852 | 4.2681 | 6.0814 | 8.6361 | 12.2236 | 17.2456 | 24.2538 | 34.0039 |
| 38 | 3.0748 | 4.4388 | 6.3855 | 9.1543 | 13.0793 | 18.6253 | 26.4367 | 37.4043 |
| 39 | 3.1670 | 4.6164 | 6.7048 | 9.7035 | 13.9948 | 20.1153 | 28.8160 | 41.1448 |
| 40 | 3.2620 | 4.8010 | 7.0400 | 10.2857 | 14.9745 | 21.7245 | 31.4094 | 45.2593 |
| 41 | 3.3599 | 4.9931 | 7.3920 | 10.9029 | 16.0227 | 23.4625 | 34.2363 | 49.7852 |
| 42 | 3.4607 | 5.1928 | 7.7616 | 11.5570 | 17.1443 | 25.3395 | 37.3175 | 54.7637 |
| 43 | 3.5645 | 5.4005 | 8.1497 | 12.2505 | 18.3444 | 27.3666 | 40.6761 | 60.2401 |
| 44 | 3.6715 | 5.6165 | 8.5572 | 12.9855 | 19.6285 | 29.5560 | 44.3370 | 66.2641 |
| 45 | 3.7816 | 5.8412 | 8.9850 | 13.7646 | 21.0025 | 31.9204 | 48.3273 | 72.8905 |
| 46 | 3.8950 | 6.0748 | 9.4343 | 14.5905 | 22.4726 | 34.4741 | 52.6767 | 80.1795 |
| 47 | 4.0119 | 6.3178 | 9.9060 | 15.4659 | 24.0457 | 37.2320 | 57.4176 | 88.1975 |
| 48 | 4.1323 | 6.5705 | 10.4013 | 16.3939 | 25.7289 | 40.2106 | 62.5852 | 97.0172 |
| 49 | 4.2562 | 6.8333 | 10.9213 | 17.3775 | 27.5299 | 43.4274 | 68.2179 | 106.7190 |
| 50 | 4.3839 | 7.1067 | 11.4674 | 18.4302 | 29.4570 | 46.9016 | 74.3575 | 117.3909 |

*Note:* 3% to 10% future value factors (compounded annually). Used to figure how much
$1 will increase at a stated percentage per year. *Example:* $100 at 5% return per year
will have a value in five years of $127.63 ($100 x 1.2763 = $127.63).

# Figure 5.5

# Future Value of $1 per Year Invested

| Years | 3% | 4% | 5% | 6% | 7% | 8% | 9% | 10% |
|---|---|---|---|---|---|---|---|---|
| 1 | 1.0300 | 1.0400 | 1.0500 | 1.0600 | 1.0700 | 1.0800 | 1.0900 | 1.1000 |
| 2 | 2.0909 | 2.1216 | 2.1525 | 2.1836 | 2.2149 | 2.2464 | 2.2781 | 2.3100 |
| 3 | 3.1836 | 3.2465 | 3.3101 | 3.3746 | 3.4399 | 3.5061 | 3.5731 | 3.6410 |
| 4 | 4.3091 | 4.4163 | 4.5256 | 4.6371 | 4.7507 | 4.8666 | 4.9847 | 5.1051 |
| 5 | 5.4684 | 5.6330 | 5.8019 | 5.9753 | 6.1533 | 6.3359 | 6.5233 | 6.7156 |
| 6 | 6.6625 | 6.8983 | 7.1420 | 7.3938 | 7.6540 | 7.9228 | 8.2004 | 8.4872 |
| 7 | 7.8923 | 8.2142 | 8.5491 | 8.8975 | 9.2598 | 9.6366 | 10.0285 | 10.4359 |
| 8 | 9.1591 | 9.5828 | 10.0266 | 10.4913 | 10.9780 | 11.4876 | 12.0210 | 12.5795 |
| 9 | 10.4639 | 11.0061 | 11.5779 | 12.1808 | 12.8164 | 13.4866 | 14.1929 | 14.3974 |
| 10 | 11.8078 | 12.4864 | 13.2068 | 13.9716 | 14.7836 | 15.6455 | 16.5603 | 17.5312 |
| 11 | 13.1920 | 14.0258 | 14.9171 | 15.8699 | 16.8885 | 17.9771 | 19.1407 | 20.3843 |
| 12 | 14.6178 | 15.6268 | 16.7130 | 17.8821 | 19.1406 | 20.4953 | 21.9534 | 23.5227 |
| 13 | 16.0863 | 17.2919 | 18.5986 | 20.0151 | 21.5505 | 23.2149 | 25.0192 | 26.9750 |
| 14 | 17.5989 | 19.0236 | 20.5786 | 22.2760 | 24.1290 | 26.1521 | 28.3609 | 30.7725 |
| 15 | 19.1569 | 20.8245 | 22.6575 | 24.6725 | 26.8881 | 29.3243 | 32.0034 | 34.9497 |
| 16 | 20.7616 | 22.6975 | 24.8404 | 27.2129 | 29.8402 | 32.7502 | 35.9737 | 39.5447 |
| 17 | 22.4144 | 24.6454 | 27.1324 | 29.9057 | 32.9990 | 36.4502 | 40.3013 | 44.5992 |
| 18 | 24.1169 | 26.6712 | 29.5390 | 32.7600 | 36.3790 | 40.4463 | 45.0185 | 50.1591 |
| 19 | 25.8704 | 28.7781 | 32.0660 | 35.7856 | 39.9955 | 44.7620 | 50.1601 | 56.2750 |
| 20 | 27.6765 | 30.9692 | 34.7193 | 38.9927 | 43.8652 | 49.4229 | 55.7645 | 63.0025 |
| 21 | 29.5368 | 33.2480 | 37.5052 | 42.3923 | 48.0057 | 54.4568 | 61.8733 | 70.4027 |
| 22 | 31.4529 | 35.6179 | 40.4305 | 45.9958 | 52.4361 | 59.8933 | 68.5319 | 78.5430 |
| 23 | 33.4265 | 38.0826 | 43.5020 | 49.8156 | 57.1767 | 65.7648 | 75.7898 | 87.4973 |
| 24 | 35.4593 | 40.6459 | 46.7271 | 53.8645 | 62.2490 | 72.1059 | 83.7009 | 97.3471 |
| 25 | 37.5530 | 43.3117 | 50.1135 | 58.1564 | 67.6765 | 78.9544 | 92.3240 | 108.1818 |
| 26 | 39.7096 | 46.0842 | 53.6691 | 62.7058 | 73.4838 | 86.3508 | 101.7231 | 120.0999 |

**Figure 5.5** *continued*

| Years | 3% | 4% | 5% | 6% | 7% | 8% | 9% | 10% |
|---|---|---|---|---|---|---|---|---|
| 27 | 41.9309 | 48.9676 | 57.4026 | 67.5281 | 79.6977 | 94.3388 | 111.9682 | 133.2099 |
| 28 | 44.2189 | 51.9663 | 61.3227 | 72.6398 | 86.3465 | 102.9659 | 123.1354 | 147.6309 |
| 29 | 46.5754 | 55.0849 | 65.4388 | 78.0582 | 93.4608 | 112.2832 | 135.3075 | 163.4940 |
| 30 | 49.0027 | 58.3283 | 69.7608 | 83.8017 | 101.0730 | 122.3459 | 148.5752 | 180.9434 |
| 31 | 51.5028 | 61.7015 | 74.2988 | 89.8898 | 109.2182 | 133.2135 | 163.0370 | 200.1378 |
| 32 | 54.0778 | 65.2095 | 79.0638 | 96.3432 | 117.9334 | 144.9506 | 178.8003 | 221.2515 |
| 33 | 56.7302 | 68.8579 | 84.0670 | 103.1838 | 127.2588 | 157.6267 | 195.9823 | 244.4767 |
| 34 | 59.4621 | 72.6522 | 89.3203 | 110.4348 | 137.2369 | 171.3168 | 214.7108 | 270.0244 |
| 35 | 62.2759 | 76.5983 | 94.8363 | 118.1209 | 147.9135 | 186.1021 | 235.1247 | 298.1268 |
| 36 | 65.1742 | 80.7022 | 100.6281 | 126.2681 | 159.3374 | 202.0703 | 257.3759 | 329.0395 |
| 37 | 68.1594 | 84.9703 | 106.7095 | 134.9042 | 171.5610 | 219.3158 | 281.6298 | 363.0434 |
| 38 | 71.2342 | 89.4091 | 113.0950 | 144.0585 | 184.6403 | 237.9412 | 308.0665 | 400.4478 |
| 39 | 74.4013 | 94.0255 | 119.7998 | 153.7620 | 198.6351 | 258.0565 | 336.8824 | 441.5926 |
| 40 | 77.6633 | 98.8265 | 126.8398 | 164.0477 | 213.6096 | 279.7810 | 368.2919 | 486.8518 |
| 41 | 81.0232 | 103.8196 | 134.2318 | 174.9505 | 229.6322 | 303.2435 | 402.5281 | 536.6370 |
| 42 | 84.4839 | 109.0124 | 141.9933 | 186.5076 | 246.7765 | 328.5830 | 439.8457 | 591.4007 |
| 43 | 88.0484 | 114.4129 | 150.1430 | 198.7580 | 265.1209 | 355.9496 | 480.5218 | 651.6408 |
| 44 | 91.7199 | 120.0294 | 158.7002 | 211.7435 | 284.7493 | 385.5056 | 524.8587 | 717.9048 |
| 45 | 95.5015 | 125.8706 | 167.6852 | 225.5081 | 305.7518 | 417.4261 | 573.1860 | 790.7953 |
| 46 | 99.3965 | 131.9454 | 177.1194 | 240.0986 | 328.2244 | 451.9002 | 625.8628 | 870.9749 |
| 47 | 103.4084 | 138.2632 | 187.0254 | 255.5645 | 352.2701 | 489.1322 | 683.2804 | 959.1723 |
| 48 | 107.5406 | 144.8337 | 197.4267 | 271.9584 | 377.9990 | 529.3427 | 745.8657 | 1056.1896 |
| 49 | 111.7969 | 151.6671 | 208.3480 | 289.3359 | 405.5289 | 572.7702 | 814.0836 | 1162.9085 |
| 50 | 116.1808 | 158.7738 | 219.8154 | 307.7561 | 434.9860 | 619.6718 | 888.4411 | 1280.2994 |

*Note:* Time value factors are used to figure what a stated amount of money will grow to per year. Future value of $1 per year (annual compounding). *Example:* $1,000 per year at 7% = $434,986 in 50 years ($1,000 x 434.986 = $434,986).

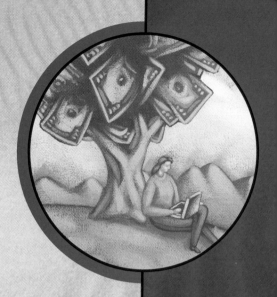

# chapter six

# Retirement Plans

I t seems as though everything in life has become more complicated over the years. This is especially true in the areas of medicine and retirement plans. Just as new techniques and equipment have greatly improved your medical skills, so have the many savings programs authorized by Congress and the IRS improved your ability to save, for each of them enables participants to set aside a certain percentage of their paychecks tax-deferred. The government's noble idea is to encourage prudent long-term investing for retirement; surely the reasoning takes into account Social Security's current troubles.

If you own your practice, this chapter will outline the positives and negatives of eight basic plans and offer guidance for implementing a retirement program to benefit both you and your employees. As an employed physician, this chapter will give you a better understanding of your employer's plan. If you are negotiating with a hospital or managed care organization, this information can help you bolster your contract and remuneration.

# IRAs

IRAs are, of course, the stand-alone individual tax-deferred program. An IRA is the place where your money should end up as rollovers from qualified plans because they are generously open and can be professionally managed and used. IRAs should be utilized by physicians who are young, in school, or anytime they qualify. You should even go so far as to use part of your school allowance to establish an IRA. Regardless of your position, an IRA is a great tool and can grow to large amounts, particularly if you can begin contributing at an early age.

While the IRS prohibits individuals older than seventy years of age from making tax-deductible IRA contributions, for semiretired physicians they may serve as a good source of tax-deferred retirement savings. IRAs of any type are open to a multitude of investment strategies; they can be easily managed, are self-directed, and don't require excessive paperwork. IRAs can be funded after the end of the given calendar year up to the time of the filing of your personal income tax return or April 15. The maximum individual yearly IRA contribution is $2,000 ($4,000 if your spouse qualifies). On the down side, a $2,000 yearly contribution is dishearteningly small. Assets are also subject to state law and, in some cases, are vulnerable to lawsuits. Whereas they may be well suited for those early in their careers and for semiretired physicians, the vast majority of physicians with moderate to significant earnings will find better tax-sheltered plans elsewhere.

# SEP Plans

SEP is an acronym for Simplified Employee Pension plan. SEPs are available to any for-profit employer, including self-employed physicians, and are reasonably easy to establish. They can also be established after the end of the calendar year, and they can be funded at any point up to the tax filing date. Another advantage is that if you establish a SEP plan, you do not have to serve as trustee (appointed to carry out the terms of a trust) or fiduciary (responsible for the handling of funds for other persons or firms). Contributions are made payable directly to the IRA accounts of both the owner and plan participants. A SEP fits conveniently between qualified plans and IRA accounts. It is a qualified plan until the contribution is deposited, at which point it becomes an IRA. SEP plans allow employers to contribute up to 15 percent of eligible compensation into their plans. The employer is responsible for covering any employee who made more than $300 in a fifty-two-week period (adjusted for inflation) and worked three out of the past five years. The IRS provides a simplified one-page form to adopt a SEP plan. The SEP is easy to understand and implement. Like an IRA, it does not require too much paperwork, and contributions are elected on a year-to-year basis.

You can contribute up to 15 percent of your eligible compensation into a SEP (for a maximum contribution of $24,000, based on a $160,000 salary). To discourage employers from manipulating their SEP plans for personal benefit, however, the contribution percentage you make for yourself must also be made for your eligible employees. Another disadvantage is that the contributions made for employees are not subject to vesting (they are 100 percent vested); this means they can be withdrawn immediately from the individual participant's IRA account after the money has been deposited. A SEP is great for self-employed physicians who have few employees. They are well suited to people who hate paperwork, want an absolute minimum of involvement with the IRS, and wish to avoid paying attorney's and administration fees.

# Profit-Sharing Plans

Profit-sharing plans have been around for a long time. While similar to SEP plans, the main difference lies in the fact that profit-sharing plans are more flexible and create a trust where employer contributions are deposited. This subjects the entire plan to the guidelines set forth by the Employee Retirement Income Security Act (ERISA) and creates other opportunities not available with SEP plans.

Because employers already pay into a retirement plan for their employees in the form of Social Security, the IRS views qualified retirement plans such as profit-sharing plans, along with Social Security, as one overall program. The IRS recognizes these Social Security payments and allows employers to benefit from their profit-sharing plans as long as the difference in benefits is attributable to Social Security. The IRS refers to this as permitted disparity. Plan administrators are able to use a revised formula that allows them to give a greater allocation to the more highly compensated employers' own profit-sharing plan. This can amount to as much as a $2,000 difference in the physician's favor on the same contribution when you compare a profit-sharing plan to a SEP plan.

An additional profit-sharing advantage is vesting (nonforfeitable right into the trust). A profit-sharing plan may require all employees to work a certain number of years (maximum of seven) before they are fully vested into the program. Those employees who leave before working the mandatory years forfeit all or part of the benefits that have been put into the trust on their behalf. After they leave, they receive a payment on the amount of money that is vested, and the balance of the money is forfeited and redistributed to the remaining participants. If your practice has any turnover at all, this vesting advantage could significantly increase your benefit in the plan as years go by. Profit-sharing plans also allow employers to make participant loans if the business entity form is a professional corporation. Loans of up to $50,000 (tax-free) can be taken out to use for liquidity needs (college education, down payments on a home, etc).

All self-employed physicians should consider a profit-sharing plan as an option. This plan doesn't lock you into contributions on a year-to-year basis, and it adds flexibility, especially for young physicians. Employers that experience moderate to high employee turnover stand to benefit from the vesting provision, which, over time, will significantly add to benefits that accrue for the employer and loyal employees.

Profit-sharing plans require an increase in paperwork and regulations to satisfy the IRS and Department of Labor. Also, because a trust is created, someone must act as trustee; this is a role typically fulfilled either by the employer or by a trust company for a fee. While using a trust company to act as a trustee may make plan sponsors feel better, it doesn't really relieve the plan sponsor of any liability. Quite often, the owner elects to become its own trustee, which allows maximum flexibility and control over plan assets. Generally, the primary down side to profit-sharing plans, as compared to a SEP, is the increased administration and regulation costs. They are best suited for young, self-employed physicians who need a flexible contribution schedule. A profit-sharing plan is not the most efficient plan for a physician whose wages are steady, who is relatively older than his or her employees, or who has done little to prepare for retirement. It allows employers to put away $30,000 or 15 percent of compensation, whichever is less.

# Money Purchase Plans

Money purchase plans are similar to profit-sharing plans in that a trust must be established, and there is a fairly high level of paperwork. The main advantage of the money purchase plan over a profit-sharing plan is that the maximum contribution formula is increased from 15 percent up to as much as 25 percent of salary. This is the maximum contribution allowed under the general category of "defined contribution plans." Defined contribution plans include profit-sharing plans, money purchase plans, and their variants such as 401k and age-weighted plans (discussed later in this chapter). They also offer the same basic features as profit-sharing plans, including forfeitures, which usually seek to reduce company contributions and participant loans. Money purchase plans can also be used in conjunction with profit-sharing plans to establish a floor/ceiling combination. Typically this design feature will have a 5 percent to 10 percent mandatory money purchase contribution and then allow for an additional profit-sharing plan contribution where there is sufficient profit to do so.

The main disadvantage of money purchase plans is that contributions at a given level (up to 25 percent) are mandatory on a year-by-year basis. The plan can be terminated, frozen, or changed after the fact, but the physician is obligated to fund at whatever level was in place at the beginning of the plan year.

Money purchase plans are recommended if you:

1. Have a stable practice.

2. Have the extra cash flow to maximize your contributions into a qualified plan.

3. Want a relatively simple approach to plan design as opposed to a defined benefit plan.

Physicians whose income varies on a year-to-year basis or who cannot make sustained contributions at a given level should not choose a money purchase plan.

## Cooking Schools from Around the World

| | |
|---|---|
| Bon Vivant School of Cooking of Seattle | 206 727-7537 |
| California Culinary Academy | 800 229-2433<br>www.baychef.com |
| Dubrulle International Culinary & Hotel Institute of Canada | 800 667-7288<br>www.dubrulle.com |
| The French Culinary Institute | 888 324-2433 |
| International Culinary Academy | 800 447-8324<br>www.computer-tech.com |
| Peter Kump's New York Cooking School | 800 522-4610 |
| La Cucina al Focalare | 800 988-2851 |
| Le Cordon Bleu Classic French Cooking School | 800 457-2433 |
| New England Culinary Institute | 877 223-6324 |
| Pacific Institute of Culinary Arts | 800 416-4040<br>www.picularts.bc.ca |
| The Restaurant School | 877 925-6884 |
| The Rhode School of Cuisine | 800 447-1311 |
| Ritz Escoffier Ecole de Gastronomie Francaise | 800 966-5758 |
| The School of the Culinary Arts | 800 543-4860 |
| Scottsdale Culinary Institute | 800 848-2433<br>www.chefs.com/culinary |
| Southern California School of Culinary Arts | 888 900-2433<br>www.scsca.com |
| Western Culinary Institute | 800 666-0312<br>www.westernculinary.com |

# 401k Plans

The 401k is always an accessory to a profit-sharing plan. If you are involved in a 401k plan, by definition you have a profit-sharing plan, and as we will see, that is important. The main distinction of a 401k plan is that it allows employees to make contributions from their paychecks on a pretax payroll basis. Employee contributions are always fully vested (recoverable) and are deposited into the trust for the benefit of the employees. Typically, the 401k plan is established so that employees have increased control over investment decisions, particularly with regard to their contributions.

401k plans theoretically shift the burden of funding from the employer to the employee. Employees can be rewarded by use of a matching system, where by employers encourage worker participation through an offer to match contributions up to a certain percentage. Employers may also be able to make additional discretionary contributions on either an integrated basis or an age-weighted basis, which we will discuss later. 401k plans are extremely complex, requiring careful and meticulous installation, administration, and communication procedures. Installing a 401k is the retirement plan equivalent of delicate heart surgery. Although anyone can establish a 401k, a skilled expert is required to bring the plan up and administer it, while keeping the plan free of trouble with complex IRS and Department of Labor regulations.

401ks are well suited to large employers with an employee base of at least twenty-five. Older, financially sophisticated employees who are part of a two-income family are the optimum members of a 401k plan. Remember, for a 401k to be successful, the concept has to be sold not only to you as the physician employer, but to each and every one of your employees. A 401k works well when employees are looking for ways to put away additional money for retirement. Not all employees are interested in this opportunity. Conversely, a 401k is not the wise choice for small practices with few employees (typically twenty-five or less). This is because the administrative costs can be very steep on a per person basis. Nor do 401ks work well for self-employed physicians who despise paperwork and are in a situation where the technical expertise is not available from an outside source to keep the plan running well.

# SIMPLE Plans

SIMPLE is one of those congressionally generated acronyms for Savings Incentive Match Plan for Employees. It comes in two varieties: 401k SIMPLE and SIMPLE IRA. They resemble the evil and outstanding twin syndrome; 401k SIMPLE is the malcontent, and SIMPLE IRA is the exceptional one.

SIMPLE allows employees to defer up to the first $6,000 of their income into their personal SIMPLE IRA account without any percentage limits. SIMPLE also puts a cap on employer cost by mandating that an employer match employee contributions up to the first 3 percent of compensation in any given three out of five years, and match employee contributions up to the first 1 percent in any given two out of five years.

Compared to other qualified retirement plans, SIMPLE lives up to its name in terms of reporting requirements involving paperwork and IRS regulations. For employers with a W-2 income of $50,000 or less and Schedule C income of $60,000 or less, SIMPLE is easily the most efficient retirement plan.

SIMPLE IRA does have disadvantages. It offers no flexibility whatsoever. It has a simple formula and a simple match with very little deviation. So SIMPLE either works or it doesn't; it can't be easily changed or manipulated in your favor. Another disadvantage is that it cannot be used in connection with any other qualified plan such as profit-sharing, defined benefit, and money purchase plans. It can, however, replace another plan once that plan is terminated.

SIMPLE was designed for small business owners with fewer than one hundred employees, whose yearly contribution goals are $12,000 or less per year. It was also designed for employers who want to limit the amount of money they are required to put in for their employees. Unlike the 401k, it works best in those situations where the employees are probably not going to participate, either because of their younger age or relatively lower pay.

SIMPLE is ideal for any individual who has income in addition to W-2 income, such as moonlighting income, or any employer who works two jobs and is self-employed at one of them. SIMPLE is also for those employers who want to give their employees something, but who want to keep it within very tight boundaries. It is not for those who want to accumulate wealth in a retirement plan quickly because allocations to a self-employed physician are limited to $12,000 a year. In addition, SIMPLE may not be appropriate for most physicians due to their high income. SIMPLE would not work well for an older physician who needs a more customized type of plan to be able to play "catch-up" on a target amount of retirement benefits.

# Age-Weighted and New Comparability Profit-Sharing Plans

These new types of plans were created by the Tax Revenue Act of 1986 and are the IRS's attempt to regulate this act. In a figurative sense, the IRS closed the front door, then opened the back door. These plans are highly favorable to self-employed physicians.

In order for these plans to work, you need either a large disparity in age (with the employer physician being much older) or multiple owners in a corporation and clear division lines between employee duties. Typically the contributions are discretionary and can be made on a year-to-year basis. The allocations can be up to $30,000 and can specify a vesting requirement. These plans can also exclude employees who leave service before year's end. They can have the other features of the aforementioned profit-sharing plan and may be used in conjunction with a 401k plan.

Much like 401ks, these plans are incredibly complex, needing a first rate administrator to keep them in compliance with IRS regulations. Therefore, for small practices they are expensive to install and administer. They also have the other disadvantages associated with profit-sharing plans. Group physician practices will find these plans ideal, especially when the age of the owner/officers is above that of the rank and file employees. Large companies like hospitals, HMOs, etc, where there are clearly segregated lines of duties, are equally well suited to them.

# Defined Benefit Plans

We tend to think of defined benefit plans (DBPs) as the smokestack plans of the early 1940s and 50s. These plans are based on a benefit at retirement rather than a year-by-year contribution. They require that an enrolled actuary be used. An enrolled actuary is certified by the IRS to determine the yearly contributions needed to keep these plans solvent.

Defined benefit plans have two efficient uses: for a large, stable practice with a long-standing workforce that wants to provide an excellent, fixed, ongoing benefit strictly for retirement purposes; and for highly compensated, older, closely held practices, with few employees and a need to accumulate significant benefits over a short time period. They offer the largest contribution tax deductions of any other type of program given an older employee. Compared to $30,000 (the largest allocation allowed in any other type of plan), employers are allowed to take up to a $90,000 deduction and allocation. But defined benefit plans are complicated, expensive, and confusing to physicians. They should not be undertaken unless you are willing to keep the plan open for a minimum of ten years. Contributions are required and may go up dramatically as you get closer to retirement and/or if you have poor investment performance.

Very few physicians should consider a defined benefit plan unless they fit into one of the two favorable categories, and even those physicians should think carefully before establishing such a program in the face of recent government regulations. However, if a DBP is for you, it will create tax-favored wealth faster than any other plan.

Figure 6.1 (Comparison of Plans for Retirement) summarizes the contribution limits, investment options, administrative requirements, and major advantages and disadvantages of each of the plans discussed above.

# Ten Worst Mistakes Regarding Retirement Plans

1. *Not doing anything because the laws seem so complicated and may change.* General Douglas MacArthur said, "There is no security in this world, only opportunity." This is certainly true in saving money on taxes and building assets toward retirement. Laws may come and go, Congress may change things, but tax-qualified retirement plans are the best vehicle to shield assets from current taxes to establish large amounts of retirement income for future years.

2. *Procrastinating.* Generally speaking, the earlier you start saving, even with a small amount, the better off you are. In my career, I have worked with scores of retirement plans and, truly, the physicians who start early reap great benefits from the magic of compound returns.

3. *Establishing a plan and then not remaining consistent about funding the plan.* Some people, on the advice of their accountant, start a flexible plan but fail to continue to fund it. As the years go by, administrative costs on the young plan all but eat away any gains that the plan experiences, leaving these persons exasperated because things have not worked out. If you are going to establish a plan, you have to be consistent with funding it.

4. *Expecting your CPA or CFP to be an expert on pension plans.* Your CPA or CFP is often the person who will tell you that the time has come to establish a plan. While the professional standing of a CPA or CFP is

**Figure 6.1**

## Comparison of Plans for Retirement

| Plan Type | Contribution Limit | Investment Options | Suitability for Employees | Administrative Requirements | Key Advantage | Key Disadvantage | Who Should Consider |
|---|---|---|---|---|---|---|---|
| **IRA** | Up to the lesser of $2,000 or 100% of earned income if eligible | Annuities, mutual funds, CDs; no life insurance | Personal plan; not designed for employee benefit purposes | None | Completely your own plan | $2,000 contribution limit | Almost everyone's "first" plan |
| **SEP** | 15% of earned income or $30,000, whichever is less | Same as IRA | Limited by restricted plan options | Simple document; no annual filing | Employee plan with least paperwork | Must include part-time employees | Employer with maximum IRA and no employees |
| **SIMPLE** | Up to first $6,000 of earned income | Same as IRA | Best for small business under $60,000 income | Document; annual meeting; some tracking | Largest deduction for owners with limited income | Must match employee contribution up to 3% | Smaller employer *with low income*; employer with side income |
| **Profit-Sharing Plan** | 15% of overall pay up to $30,000 individually | Any prudent investment, including life insurance | Very good for work incentive; appeals to younger employees | Document; annual government filing; employee reports | Flexible contributions | Provides limited benefits for older participants | Employer with young employees and variable income |
| **Age-Weighted Plan** | 15% of overall pay up to $30,000 individually | Any prudent investment, including life insurance | Appeals to older owners and officers | Document; annual government filing; employee reports | Flexible contributions and high allocation to older worker | High installation costs | Older owner of closely held company |

**Figure 6.1** *continued*

| Plan Type | Contribution Limit | Investment Options | Suitability for Employees | Administrative Requirements | Key Advantage | Key Disadvantage | Who Should Consider |
|---|---|---|---|---|---|---|---|
| **New Comparability Plan** | 15% of overall pay up to $30,000 individually | Any prudent investment, including life insurance | Appeals to older owners who have younger partners | Document; annual government filing; employee reports | Flexible contributions and high allocation to older worker | High installation and administration costs | Multiple owners of closely held company |
| **401k** | $9,500 in employee contributions up to 15% overall | Any prudent investment, including life insurance | Best for younger employees if maximum contribution made | Document; annual government filing; employee reports | Employee investment direction; positive employee perception | Complex administrative requirements | Larger, stable company that wants to retain employees |
| **Money Purchase Plan** | 25% of pay or $30,000, whichever is less | Same as profit-sharing | Best for younger employees if maximum contribution made | Same as profit-sharing | Larger contribution limit than other defined benefit plans | No contribution flexibility | Employer with young employees and stable income |
| **Defined Benefit Plan** | Maximum benefit is 100% of pay up to $125,000 | Same as profit-sharing | Best for older employees due to guaranteed benefit | Same as profit-sharing, plus actuarial certification | Favors older participants | Complex administrative requirements | Older employer with stable income |

very noteworthy, neither CPAs nor CFPs are usually experts on the technical requirements involved in pension plans, or even the right people to recommend the best type of plan or to keep the plan in compliance. Unless he or she hails from a very big firm with a specific department in this area, your CPA, CFP, or accountant is not set up to handle this kind of work. Ask your CPA or CFP for a referral to a good, fee-only retirement plan design and administration firm.

5. *Keeping your employees in the dark about their interest in the plan.* First of all, this is illegal. If you are caught, the Department of Labor (DOL) can levy heavy fines and the IRS can disallow the plan. Second, it really does not make much sense because if the plan is properly explained, even if it is a plan that is favorable to the owner, the employees are going to feel that at least something is being done on their behalf. Don't mislead your employees. Use the plan as a tool to make your employees feel good about working for you.

6. *Choosing the wrong type of plan based on bad advice.* This comes from the cookie cutter approach that many broker-dealers, insurance agents, and banks employ. Employers are set up with 401k plans because that type of plan is most beneficial to the broker-dealer, not the client. When a plan is recommended out of convenience rather than what is best in a given situation, its efficiency is drastically reduced.

7. *Attempting to be your own investment manager.* ERISA requires that if you are a plan administrator, sponsor, or trustee, you must act in a prudent manner. This usually means hiring a registered investment advisor who manages your portfolio under established goals and constraints. If you're going to manage your own IRAs or TSAs, consider the do-it-yourself portfolios showcased in chapter eight and utilize mutual funds for long-term performance.

8. *Letting an investment (product) seller guide your plan.* Brokers, insurance agents, and other commission receivers are usually too caught up in the allure of big commissions to objectively guide your plan. A person that recommends an annuity to fund your plan (unless it's a TIAA/CREF) may be after a commission, and their advice should be avoided. Wrap accounts, especially those using mutual funds, are very expensive and often have layers of hidden, unnecessary fees. Find a good fee-only registered investment advisor or use the do-it-yourself portfolio strategy.

9. *Running afoul of IRS regulations by not taking seriously the issue of plan administration.* Every qualified plan must identify a named plan administrator. The plan administrator is responsible to the IRS and the DOL for different compliance issues within the plan. Should you decide

to undertake this role, remember your potential liability to plan participants is nothing compared to your potential liability to the IRS and the
DOL. There are banks and trust companies who will take on the duties
of trustee, but there are not many firms that will assign themselves
directly as plan administrator. The laws are much too complex for
physicians, or anyone else who is not directly in the business, to administer their plan. You need the services of a contract administrator or a
third-party administrator (on a fee basis) to keep the plan on track.

10. *Choosing to stay ignorant about your plan.* In a nutshell, here are five
key issues to be aware of:

    a. Your plan document will need to be updated regularly (usually every
    four years).

    b. In some cases, you will need to file an annual report with the IRS
    about your plan (5500 series).

    c. You must provide information to your employees each year about the
    plan.

    d. You should review your plan's investment performance with your
    investment advisor at least once a year.

    e. You should know the names and duties of each of the individuals
    involved in your plan, including: trustee, plan administrator, plan
    sponsor, investment advisor, and contract administrator.

Navigating through the details of each retirement plan can be overwhelm-
ing. Don't get discouraged. A competent, fee-only financial advisor should
be able to quickly guide you to the right plan.

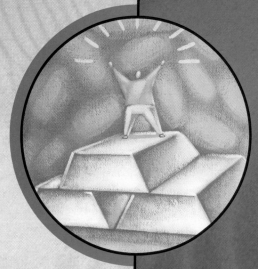

# chapter seven

# Invest Wisely

**A**s the value of your retirement plan starts to build, you will become increasingly aware of the importance of controlling the risks and rewards of investing. Investments are the tools to help you build retirement security. Your investment goal should be twofold: (1) to accumulate sufficient assets to retire and, (2) to ensure that your retirement portfolio will provide you with lifetime (your whole life) income security. This is no small task to ask of your accumulated wealth. Inflation, depressions, stock market manias, real estate crashes, bond defaults, wars, and bear markets are the pesky land mines that will affect your portfolio's real (after taxes and inflation) return. Still, investments, if used properly, provide an incredible opportunity to build assets and achieve your retirement goals.

# Stocks

First we need to discuss reality. The fabulous stock market performance of the last ten years (1989–1999) is not reality. Realistically, you cannot assume returns of 18 percent to 25 percent per year, or even 10 percent per year, in your retirement projections. Until the recent unprecedented returns of the Dow Jones Industrial Average and Standard & Poor's 500 index, the stock market grew much like the economy and returned approximately 10 percent per year (approximately 5 percent from dividends and 5 percent from capital gains). Some years it lost 43 percent; other years it made over 50 percent; but over time it has returned in real money (after inflation) 7 percent.

History has shown that it is silly to assume stock market returns in excess of historic averages. If you added the last ten years' performance of the stock market to historic sixty-year averages, you could conclude that the real inflation-adjusted return of the stock market was 9 percent. A 7 percent return over time is more accurate and a better number for keeping your portfolio on track. The reality is that all you can do is make sure that your portfolio is managed in a way that is consistent with your risk tolerance and financial needs.

Stocks must be considered in the construction of any long-term-oriented investment strategy in order to optimize potential

> **The average fee-only financial advisor serving physicians found that . . .**
> Their average client under age 40 has $100,000 to $200,000 in retirement investments. Those ages 40 to 50 have $350,000 to $750,000, while those not yet retired but over age 50 have $750,000 to $2 million.

growth, but your portfolio should also allow you to sleep at night. In evaluating stocks and most other investments, you must evaluate risk. Risk can be minimized by using various tools of investing such as asset allocation, diversification, security analysis, and active management.

If you own volatile investments such as stocks and understand their positive characteristics (dividends, appreciation, long-term performance) and negative ones (volatility, business risk), your portfolio can be structured to succeed if it utilizes a diversified portfolio of carefully selected bargain investments. Stocks can be a part of those investments.

Let's look at stocks and the stock market objectively. Stocks can represent ownership of a portfolio of US government bonds, a company trying to turn lead into gold, or stocks owning stocks. Mutual funds are a type of stock that can own stocks.

When most people think of investing in stocks, they think of owning interest in a corporation such as Merck. They hope that Merck will grow, increase dividends, and prosper throughout the years. When you invest in common stocks, such as Merck, you own something. You can choose to invest in companies that are big and well established, or companies that you hope will grow big in the future. However, the most important criterion in evaluating stocks and other investments is evaluating risk. Remember that all investments have risk; it cannot be avoided when you choose to invest. As a reward for bearing risk, an investor—with a well-constructed portfolio utilizing tools for lowering risk—should realize a favorable return.

As mentioned, all stocks are not created equal. There are equity investments that include stocks and other "ownership" investments that can be made all over the world in many different industries. Of course, some industries are more stable, like electric utilities, food companies, and well-diversified pharmaceuticals; and some are very unpredictable, like biotech, Internet, and information science companies. It is my sincere belief that favorable risk-adjusted returns can be achieved without undue risk by carefully researching undervalued equity investments and including them in a well-diversified portfolio. History has rewarded those investors who combined hard work, diligent study, and a disciplined approach. Due to their favorable rate of return over time, stocks should be emphasized all through the life cycle of your portfolio. This does not mean that your portfolio should be 100 percent in equities all the time so that you are forced to ride out every cycle. The idea is that your portfolio should emphasize stocks when they are undervalued and avoid them when they are expensive.

A number of physicians have mentioned the following creative formula for determining their asset allocation: subtract your age from one hundred, and the remaining number equals the percentage of your portfolio's assets you should place in the stock market. For example, if you are seventy-two, 28 percent of your assets belong in stocks (100 − 72 = 28). While handy and easy to get excited about, this formula is truly silly. Stocks as an asset class should be owned when they are bargains, based on dividend yield, price-earnings ratio, price-to-book ratio, growth prospects, etc, regardless of your age. Once you are retired and begin to construct a retirement income portfolio, you should favor more predictable income-oriented equities like utility stocks, real-estate investment trusts, convertible preferred stocks, and convertible bonds. A retirement portfolio should earn through dividends and interest at least 80 percent of what it pays out as income.

# Dividend Yields

Stock dividend yields near 3 percent or lower strongly suggest a high-risk, expensive stock market, whereas dividend yields near or above 5 percent point toward lower risk and bargain stock prices ahead. In order to keep your portfolio up-to-date and appropriately invested for tomorrow, you must open your mind and always try to purchase assets that appear undervalued. A sound strategy must balance the financial risks of investing with the opportunity that is created by these risks. As illustrated in Figures 7.1 (Dividends in History) and 7.2 (S&P 500 Dividend Yield and Future Stock Market Performance), dividend yields are one way of finding bargains and anticipating downturns in the market.

We live in a vastly different world than that of our parents and grandparents, one that requires an investment strategy that is flexible with the times. The stock markets throughout the world (combined) are now much larger than the US markets, and with today's technology it is easier to find opportunities beyond the borders of this country.

Newly industrialized countries in the Pacific Basin are now able to compete with the United States on quality, price, and delivery of goods, whereas twenty-five years ago, only the United States and a few other countries were players. Other parts of the world to watch are the huge markets and burgeoning economies in eastern Europe, South America, Africa, Russia, and China. The smart investment money today is on companies that are globally oriented. Because the United States represents only 6 percent of our world population, we must pay serious attention to the rapidly developing world economy.

## Figure 7.1

# Dividends in History

| Date | S&P 500 Dividend Yield | S&P 500 Change |
|------|------------------------|----------------|
| August 31,1929 | 2.87% | −59.2% over 21 months |
| May 31,1946 | 3.55 | −30.1% over 19 months |
| March 31, 1961 | 2.98 | −20.0% over 15 months |
| January 5, 1973 | 2.96 | −43.0% over 22 months |
| August 25, 1987 | 2.78 | −33.0% over 3 1/2 months |
| July 16, 1990 | 3.28 | −19.0% over 3 months |

*Note:* Dividend yields throughout history have been a good indicator of future stock market performance.

## Figure 7.2

# S&P 500 Dividend Yield and Future Stock Market Performance

| S&P 500 Yield | 6 Months | 1 Year | 2 Years | 3 Years |
|---------------|----------|--------|---------|---------|
| Below 3% | −1% | −5% | −10% | −1% |
| 3% to 4% | +1% | +4% | +9% | +12% |
| 4% to 5% | +7% | +14% | +21% | +26% |
| 5% to 6% | +4% | +11% | +33% | +56% |
| 6% to 7% | +6% | +12% | +32% | +45% |
| Above 7% | +8% | +29% | +42% | +63% |

Reprinted through the courtesy of the Editors of Market Logic. Copyright 1997. The Institute for Econometric Research, 2200 SW 10th St, Deerfield Beach, FL, 33442. Subscribers: 800 442-9000.

# Perception and Reality

A perfect investment does not exist for all investment cycles—that's the reality. The key to long-term investment performance is a strategy designed to provide favorable returns consistently, all the while staying true to an investment management philosophy. Figure 7.3 is the management philosophy we adopted at my firm. Use it as a guide when constructing your own investment philosophy statement or when hiring a fee-only registered investment advisor.

All investment advisors will have biases; some will stay true to the holy grail of asset allocation, others are growth oriented, and a fair number emphasize risk-adjusted bargain investments. These latter managers are often called "value" managers. In order for an investment to achieve bargain status, perception and reality must be out of sync. For example, in the 1980s the perception was that Japan was an unstoppable economic powerhouse. The reality is that those very characteristics that helped shape Japan's booming economy proceeded to become the root of her downturn. Investors who grew skeptical when Japanese stocks became three to ten times more expensive based on earnings, dividend yields, and price-to-book ratios than similar companies in the United States or Europe were well rewarded.

Many investors believe that the US stock market deserves to have its large multinational companies priced at two to three times more than smaller, similar US companies and multinational companies in other countries. Twenty years ago the opposite perception was considered reality. Large US companies were then considered stodgy, boring dinosaurs with limited growth prospects, while smaller competitors were considered smart and nimble racehorses that competed successfully by taking over market niches and grabbing market share from their larger counterparts.

Favoring bargain investments based on an analysis of their growth prospects, earnings yield, competitive factors, balance sheet analysis, products and product strategy, and relative value to other investments regardless of size has proved to be a successful long-term strategy. Figure 7.4 (Perception and Reality) can be used to help you cover many of the key issues in selecting stocks to add to your portfolio. The goal is to buy solid companies with great products and great management at the right price.

Yet too many investors try to oversimplify the complicated business of investing. Investments must be purchased and managed with foresight and understanding of the financial markets. Most often this is best accomplished by hiring experienced professionals. If you don't wish to hire a fee-only investment advisor, make a point not to trust your portfolio to stockbrokers, insurance agents, or commissioned salespeople. Instead, do it yourself under the strategy outlined in chapter eight.

**Figure 7.3**

# Investment Philosophy

## Financial & Investment Management Group, Ltd

### Our Investment Philosophy Is Based upon the Following Belief System

We believe in the following:

1. That a perfect investment does not exist for all investment cycles and that to reduce risk, assets should be reallocated to avoid overvalued assets and favor undervalued assets accordingly during each financial cycle. Thus, we believe in active portfolio management.

2. That it is important for a money manager to discipline himself to remain flexible and creative. At Financial & Investment Management Group, Ltd (FIMG), we use both fundamental and technical analyses in making our investment and asset allocation decisions.

3. That diversification should be used carefully to reduce risks and increase rewards by allocating investment portfolios as follows:

   a. Among asset classes (ie, stocks, bonds, money market funds, etc).

   b. Within each asset class, through owning many different investments within each asset class or through the use of diversified companies, mutual funds, annuities, or other investments with built-in diversification.

   c. Through management style, by utilizing outside advisors to assist in making investment and asset allocation decisions.

   d. Globally, through exploring investment opportunities worldwide.

4. That patience and perseverance are essential qualities of a money manager. A successful investor must keep a long-term horizon and avoid getting caught up in the mania of the markets. This mania is caused by rapid changes in investor psychology due to real or perceived economic, societal, or financial events.

5. That during certain periods in the market it is wiser to emphasize capital preservation, while during other periods greater emphasis must be placed on capital growth. At all times, a manager should carefully search the world for risk-adjusted bargain investments for client portfolios.

6. That it is important for a money manager to minimize all costs associated with investing. FIMG achieves this by trading at substantially discounted commissions, using no-load funds with low expense ratios, and allocating trades to brokers specializing in certain investment areas.

7. That to be totally objective, a money manager must be compensated only on a fee basis. No commissions or any other transaction-related remuneration should be received by the manager. FIMG is strictly a fee-only manager.

**Figure 7.3** *continued*

8. That a money manager should have the training, temperament, experience, and resources available that will promote success in their field. A manager "must manage," enjoy the process of management, and have passion, commitment, and love for the investment business.

9. That money managers making specific investment decisions regarding client portfolios should be accessible to their clients to discuss strategy, market outlook, conditions, and so on.

10. That our primary goal is to maintain the highest degree of integrity, ethics, and quality in working with our clients, employees, business partners, and service providers.

11. In client confidentiality and a firm "no exceptions" policy stating that no information will be sold or shared with anyone, except as required by law or with the clients' express permission.

This is the philosophy of Financial & Investment Management Group, Ltd. We believe that if you find this makes sound investment sense, then you will consider us as your investment manager.

**Figure 7.4**

# Perception and Reality

- Stocks get overvalued to an extreme.

- Stocks get undervalued to an extreme.

- Find bargains to buy when perception is different from reality.

**Your first goal is to make money:**

- Buy undervalued, bargain stocks with good prospects.

- Company's balance sheet is good.

- Company's price-to-cash flow is favorable.

- Company's cash flow is good or improving.

- Competitive forces are understood and reasonable.

- Company's earnings are good and/or improving.

- Company's management is experienced and savvy.

- Company's price-to-earnings ratio is at less than its expected growth rate.

**Your second goal is to keep from losing money by selling and/or avoiding overvalued, expensive stocks:**

- Is the company's price-to-sales, price-to-earnings, price-to-book ratio excessive when compared to its expected future growth rate?

- Is the company creating a market for competitors to enter that will lower growth and profit margins?

*Note:* Big returns are made by buying out-of-favor or misunderstood investments at bargain prices (when perception is different from reality) to make money *and by avoiding overvalued (usually) in-favor investments to keep from losing money.*

# The "Sort of" Whole Truth about Investment Management Fees

You get what you pay for—but often, you can get what you pay for, for a whole lot less!

## What is a reasonable fee?

|  | Total Fee for Management* | Commissions, etc* |
|---|---|---|
| S&P 100 Index and other indexed portfolios | 1/4%–1/2% | 1/10th of 1% |
| Actively managed US equity portfolios $1 million+ | 6/10%–1 1/4% | 1/4%–4/10% |
| Actively managed global equity portfolios $1 million+ | 3/4%–1 1/2% | 1/4%–1/2% |

\* Per year.

Investment management fees are only one component of hiring a good fee-only investment advisor, albeit a very important one. The above fees are ranges that in my opinion are reasonable. Expect to pay more for active management of small cap and global management styles, less for large cap or passive management.

# chapter eight

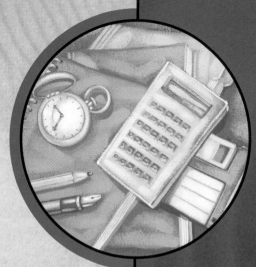

# Do-It-Yourself Portfolio Management

I f you are unable or unwilling to hire a good fee-only investment advisor with a style consistent with what feels comfortable to you, you should consider assuming the task yourself using a disciplined strategy that emphasizes no-load mutual funds. This chapter will teach you how to construct a mutual fund portfolio designed to ensure that your portfolio will provide you with reasonable and consistent returns over time.

Historically, the stock market tends to rise powerfully, only to settle back into a neutral state of balance, followed by a downturn, then a general reversal of the process. In fact, a great tool is available to measure and quantify the stock market cycles: follow the dividend yields. The variations in yields that the stock market has paid have been a solid indication of when to be in the market and when to stay on the sidelines.

A very inexpensive stock market presents itself when dividend yields inch up over 5 percent. Conversely, when yields fall below 2 percent or 3 percent, it's time to get defensive and sell. This rule is a time-tested way to gauge the market and manage a portfolio. In order to stay current and appropriately invested for tomorrow, you must always try to purchase assets that appear undervalued. Your strategy should balance the financial risks and opportunity that are created by market volatility and cycles.

# Managing Money Takes Skill

Whether you are personally up to the care and attention required to manage your own portfolio is a crucial issue. Discipline, creativity, patience, decisiveness, and steady hands in the throes of market volatility—when it's your money on the line—are some of the skills needed to achieve success. Fortunately, you can delegate a large part of your investment management to a fee-only professional if you wish or, if you do the job yourself, you might be best served to limit investment choices to a handful of carefully selected no-load mutual funds. Professionals will be much more active. They have the time and skills to research a world's worth of opportunity, from technology stocks to energy, socially responsible companies to short-term bonds, and others.

Whichever method you choose, remember that you are responsible for your investment success. Figure 8.1 (Retirement Portfolio Management Process) diagrams the interrelated steps you will need to take as part of your investment management process. Do not place your financial security totally in

## Figure 8.1

# Retirement Portfolio Management Process

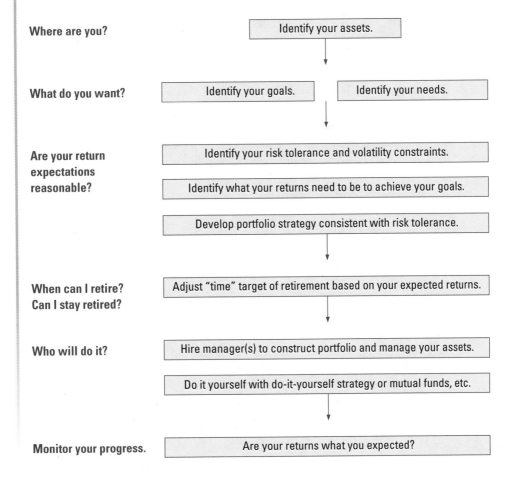

**Where are you?**   Identify your assets.

**What do you want?**   Identify your goals.   Identify your needs.

**Are your return expectations reasonable?**
Identify your risk tolerance and volatility constraints.
Identify what your returns need to be to achieve your goals.
Develop portfolio strategy consistent with risk tolerance.

**When can I retire? Can I stay retired?**
Adjust "time" target of retirement based on your expected returns.

**Who will do it?**
Hire manager(s) to construct portfolio and manage your assets.
Do it yourself with do-it-yourself strategy or mutual funds, etc.

**Monitor your progress.**   Are your returns what you expected?

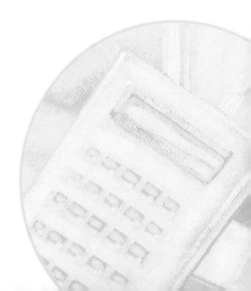

the hands of a manager, mutual funds, an intuitive friend, or anyone but yourself. Delegating this responsibility to a good fee-only manager with experience is fine and advisable, but you are still required to monitor that person and ensure that they are skillfully managing your portfolio consistent with your risk tolerance and goals.

In managing the risk of investments, the primary goal should be to avoid purchasing assets whose prices are significantly overvalued due to manias. John Maynard Keynes became very wealthy by understanding how important psychology is in determining investment values. When describing money managers in his book *The General Theory of Employment Interest Rates and Money,* he said, "They are concerned not with what the investment is really worth to a man who buys it (for keeps) but with what the market will value it under the influence of mass psychology."* Any investment strategy should emphasize utilizing manias to your benefit.

A self-managed portfolio of mutual funds should earn enough to keep pace with inflation while minimizing risk and optimizing your chances of attaining your goals. Figure 8.2 (Do-It-Yourself Strategy) details investor types and dividend yields to give an overall picture of how to proceed as a do-it-yourself investor.

In structuring a portfolio (or in hiring a money manager) you first need to address your risk tolerance. Investment strategies should be flexible and designed to capitalize on each cycle. If the market plunges from ten thousand on the Dow to six thousand, the fact that the stock market is selling at half price does not mean that you can handle more risk; nothing guarantees that the market won't fall another 50 percent. Probability and statistics surely suggest that there is less risk, yet a person's risk tolerance remains unchanged. You must trust your strategy and not sell out at the bottoms and buy at the tops.

Markets have (at extremes) reached dividend yields of over 7 percent and under 2 percent. Thus, under the do-it-yourself market cycle strategy (see the worksheets found in the appendix at the back of this book), you might buy at a yield of 5 percent and see your portfolio decreasing in value to reach a 7 percent dividend yield. Conversely, if you sell at a 3 percent yield, it doesn't mean the markets won't go down to 2 percent. Be patient and stick to your strategy.

---

* John Maynard Keynes, *The General Theory of Employment Interest Rates and Money* (New York: Harcout Brace Jovanovich, 1936).

## Figure 8.2

# Do-It-Yourself Strategy

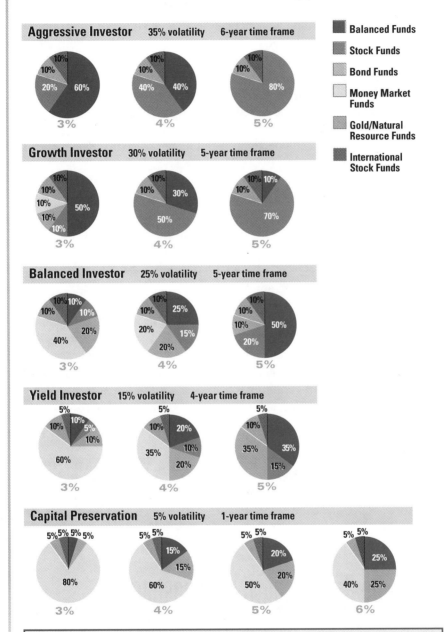

**Aggressive Investor**   35% volatility   6-year time frame

**Growth Investor**   30% volatility   5-year time frame

**Balanced Investor**   25% volatility   5-year time frame

**Yield Investor**   15% volatility   4-year time frame

**Capital Preservation**   5% volatility   1-year time frame

Legend:
- Balanced Funds
- Stock Funds
- Bond Funds
- Money Market Funds
- Gold/Natural Resource Funds
- International Stock Funds

1.  Look up your investor type (based on willingness to take risk).

2.  Consult a financial newspaper to look up the dividend yield—the pie chart gives the recommended percentages to diversify your portfolio.

3.  A list of socially responsible mutual funds and discount brokers is found at the end of this chapter. Worksheets to help monitor your portfolio are contained in the Investor Resources appendix at the back of this book.

# Enhancing Purchasing Power

The crucial decision each investor must make is how much pain or volatility is tolerable. If you trust the management technique and your $1 million portfolio loses 10 percent of its value, is that tolerable? What about 20 percent? Everyone has a threshold, even money managers. The greater the volatility that you are willing to accept, the greater the time commitment to that portfolio strategy and the greater your need for patience. The do-it-yourself strategy is structured to reward you if you can tolerate some risk and volatility to your portfolio. For example, a portfolio that can handle 25 percent volatility should do significantly better over time than a portfolio that can handle only 5 percent volatility.

The goal in investing is to enhance your purchasing power (versus inflation) consistent with your tolerance for risk. You must decide how much variability of return you can handle. This is a difficult and elusive concept, one that requires investor maturity. Quite often we don't know how much volatility we can handle. If you believe you can tolerate only 5 percent volatility (a potential 5 percent loss) over a three- to five-year period, then you would be considered a risk-averse or volatility-averse investor. If you can tolerate 35 percent to 40 percent volatility to your portfolio, your risk tolerance is very high (you can handle a tremendous amount of variability of return). With this high risk tolerance you could expect much better performance over time as long as you are patient and committed to a strategy that rewards patience. Keep in mind that the greater the volatility you are willing to accept, the greater the need for patience and time commitment.

> **The average fee-only financial advisor serving physicians found that . . .**
> Physician clients under age 40 have 60 percent to 100 percent of their retirement portfolios in equities; those over age 40 but before retirement have 45 percent to 85 percent in equities; and retirees have 30 percent to 60 percent in stocks.

# Stocks Can Be Great Long-Term Investments

The main problem with stocks is that they fluctuate in value. They would be a wonderful investment if their value only increased. Despite their volatility, over time stocks have proved to be one of the best investment classes. There has never been a twenty-five-year period where stocks have given a return of less than 3 percent. The average over most twenty-five-year periods has been a 10 percent return per year (which is about 7 percent more than inflation over the same time period). Stocks, however, do become significantly overvalued at times. This was true in 1929 and the period preceding the significant bear markets of 1973, 1974, and 1987.

Figure 8.3 (Average Annual Stock Market Returns, 1926–1998) illustrates how patience can be very rewarding. For example, the stock market's best twenty-year period is a positive 16.7 percent compounded return. The worst twenty-year period is a positive 3 percent return. The poorest ten-year period lost 1 percent a year, while the best ten-year period showed a 20 percent increase yearly. The best and worst five-year period lost 11.9 percent per year and increased 23.9 percent a year, while the one-year numbers are –43.1 percent and +55.1 percent.

Stocks, which are a very volatile asset class, favor investors with patience. Your money, however, needs to be wisely managed to ensure that it always works as hard as possible for you. Take the initiative to develop an investment strategy that offers you a good chance of success over time. There are no guarantees. Risk can be measured only by the past, yet it exists only in the future. The notion that you can develop a strategy based specifically on historical correlation and historical data is as foolish as the notion of those who believed that the moon is made of Havarti.

# Do-It-Yourself Rules

The best investments for do-it-yourself investors, to minimize risk and maximize returns, is to use a managed portfolio of diversified mutual funds, trusts, bonds, and stocks (choose companies that are well diversified in business makeup and socially responsible if you are so inclined). Mutual funds as investment tools are best suited for individuals reluctant to use an individual portfolio manager, and they are effective for any portfolio amount between $1,000 and $500,000. Hiring a fee-only (socially conscious, if you wish) professional money manager when investing amounts over $250,000 can be more cost effective than mutual funds, but make sure you hire a professional who prices his or her services competitively.

The goal of active management is to reduce the volatility on the downside. The do-it-yourself strategy emphasizes risk reduction. As assets become significantly overvalued, you sell. To increase wealth coming out of a period where the stock market has performed very poorly, you buy. As mentioned earlier, stocks historically have not done well following periods where the dividend yield on the Dow Jones or the S&P 500 has averaged under 3 percent. On the other hand, stocks have performed incredibly well when their yields have been over 5 percent. The do-it-yourself strategy uses

**Figure 8.3**

# Average Annual Stock Market Returns (1926–1998)

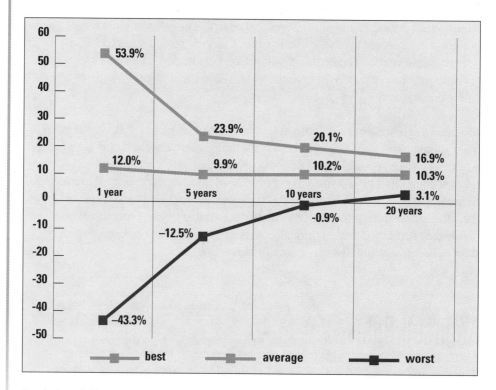

*Note:* In the period from 1926 to 1998, stocks have provided an average annual total return (capital appreciation plus dividend income) in excess of 10%. The return in individual years has varied from a low of –43.3% to a high of +53.9%, reflecting the short-term volatility of stock prices. While the average return can be used as a guide for setting expectations for future stock market returns, it may not be useful for forecasting future returns in any particular period, as stock returns are quite volatile from year to year.

*Source:* Ned Davis Research (S&P 500).

only the dividend yield as a bellwether to rebalancing your portfolio.
To reiterate, the do-it-yourself strategy expects you to follow five rules:

1. Use mutual funds or diversified trust funds.

2. Conclusively decide what portfolio strategy you wish to commit to for
   the stated period.

3. Review periodically what the yield is on the Dow Jones Industrial
   Average or the S&P 500 average.

4. Never put more than 5 percent of your assets into any one investment
   unless you choose a very well-diversified mutual fund.

5. Review your portfolio quarterly.

The do-it-yourself strategy also requires that you modify your portfolio if
dividend yields fall or rise, and that you be particularly responsive while
dividend yields are moving one way or the other (either coming up from
3 percent or down from 5 percent).

Dividend yields tend to change very slowly over time; however, if the stock
market suddenly drops 30 percent in one day, you should check your yields.
Similarly, if the stock market seems to march ahead (upwards) day after day
and the last time you checked the yields they were at 3.5 percent, it is probably a good idea to find out whether the dividend yield has crossed the 3 percent threshold again. Using history as a guide, this portfolio strategy should
not require you to rebalance your portfolio more than once or twice a year.

It is very important that once you decide on a strategy, you stick to it for at
least five years. Stay committed, even when you are pressured by friends
and business acquaintances. If you want to speculate or have some pet
investments, it's best to set aside 80 percent to 90 percent of your nest
egg in a do-it-yourself portfolio and then play with the other 10 percent to
20 percent. It is very appropriate (and smart) to have your portfolio cri-
tiqued by other professional money managers. If you own a lot of mutual
funds, have your individual funds reviewed by someone familiar with them,
and get their recommendations in writing.

When you carry out a portfolio review, I recommend hiring a fee-only
money manager who will take the time to make sure that your portfolio is
consistent with your goals and adheres to an appropriate strategy. You may
also be well served by asking them to read this book. Review the investments in your portfolio on a quarterly basis to see whether they have performed in the ballpark of similar mutual fund types. For example, if you
have three balanced mutual funds in your portfolio and one paid you an

average of 10 percent for the last twelve months, one paid 15 percent, and the last 2 percent, you should first address the poorest-performing fund to find out why it is not delivering up to expectations. Don't hesitate to call the mutual fund or review their annual or quarterly report to find the answer. Consider replacing the fund if their ideologies have changed. If you find the fund has been investing inappropriately, put it on the deathwatch, and when you need to rebalance your portfolio, replace that fund first. But don't replace it simply because it had a bad quarter or year.

During your quarterly mutual fund review, check to make sure the same company (and individuals) is still managing your portfolio. Also, check to see that their fees and investment goals have not changed over the last few months. If anything is different, you may want to consider selling that particular fund and moving your money to another fund of the same type. Most mutual funds are extremely diversified and generally follow the 5 percent rule (no more than 5 percent of assets are placed in one security or investment). Knowing this, I am still biased toward having no more than 10 percent of my money in any one growth fund, period.

# Control Your Investment Costs

I am partial to working with a discount brokerage firm specializing in diversified portfolios (stocks, bonds, mutual funds, CDs, treasury bills, etc), or with a bank or trust company that will allow you to have a diversified portfolio at a minimum cost. In my practice, we use an SIPC-insured discount brokerage company that allows us flexibility and charges low commissions. Low commission rates (when purchasing securities) and no-load mutual funds minimize the cost associated with investing and maximize your returns. If you can reduce your fee costs by even 1 percent, for example, using no-load mutual funds and avoiding high brokerage commissions or high trust company fees, it translates into money that will help offset inflation and increase your financial security.

Included at the end of this chapter is a handful of discount brokers that are:

1. SIPC-insured;

2. regulated by the New York Stock Exchange and other major exchanges; and

3. carry insurance in excess of $500,000 per portfolio.

This is the short list of my criteria for safe brokers. To choose a broker who is appropriate, I suggest you send the letter represented in Figure 8.4

**Figure 8.4**

# Evaluation Letter to Account Broker

Dear (name of broker):

I am considering setting up an account with your company, and will use predominantly open- and closed-end mutual funds to construct my portfolio. Will you allow me to buy no-load mutual funds? (Send me a list of those funds.)

What load mutual funds will you hold in my account on my behalf if I already own some?

Can I buy individually listed stocks, bonds, CDs, etc? What money market fund do you automatically invest my cash balance in?

Do you have no-transaction-fee funds (NTF)? If so, send me details. Please send me a letter addressing the above questions. In addition, I would also like to have verification that you are a member of the Securities Investors Protection Corporation and members of a stock exchange and thus regulated by their rules and regulations. Please send me your corporation's latest annual report and latest quarterly report. I'd like to receive every quarterly and annual report from your company so that I can monitor your company's financial strength.

In your letter, please outline your confidentiality safeguards, and state that you will not sell my name to anyone for solicitation of investment products or other services.

In your new investor packet, please include the following:

1. A commission schedule so that I can get an accurate idea of what it will cost to transact business through your company.

2. The name of a contact person that I may call to get more information.

3. A sample copy of your monthly portfolio statements. Will you list all my mutual funds on my monthly statement, in addition to my other assets?

I'm interested in having a relationship with you only if you will hold all my investment assets in a street name or master account.

In addition, will your company allow me check-writing privileges on my nonretirement portfolio? Can you issue a VISA debit card or other debit card? What are the costs of each of these?

Thank you for your earliest attention to the above.
Sincerely,
(Prospective Account Holder)

(Evaluation Letter to Account Broker). If you're retired, you will need to find out whether the broker will send you monthly checks and if that service is free. If it's a personal account and registered in your own name or a trust, you'll also want to know if they allow you to access that account:

1. by writing checks;

2. through a VISA debit card; or

3. via monthly checks mailed to you.

Find out the cost of these services. My bias toward discount brokers stems from the fact that many commission-oriented brokers tend to solicit you for business and can often get you off track or away from your safety-first portfolio. Usually they do this at your weakest point. It may be when your portfolio has underperformed for a few quarters and you're plainly frustrated. Discount brokers, on the other hand, simply execute your orders. Due to the increasingly competitive nature of the industry, most of them continue to offer new products and surprisingly good service at a fraction of what the full-service brokers cost.

# Managing Your Cash

Busy investors need a simple, efficient, convenient place for safekeeping their assets. Many brokerage firms, and a few bank trust departments, have responded to this need by establishing central asset management accounts, often called cash management accounts (CMAs) or financial management accounts. Some accounts will allow you to margin your securities if you need quick cash and don't want to sell your investments. They will also send you a tax summary at year-end listing all of your tax information to facilitate filing your tax return. As mentioned earlier, some of the major brokerage firms have CMAs, though I find them inconvenient and expensive for the do-it-yourself investor or the investor who uses a professional money manager. Conventional brokers often charge high fees and commissions for such services, while restricting your use of mutual funds. In addition, these brokerage firms often employ salespeople pitching new investment products, which can distract you from your investment goals. Remember, brokerage firms make money by developing and selling new products; you must decide your own strategy and stick to it. These sales calls can disrupt your long-term financial security.

# Mutual Funds

The trillion-dollar mutual fund industry has done wonders for individual investors. Mutual funds add a tremendous amount of efficiency and leverage, while reducing risk and offering professional management. Their popularity, however, has created a difficult problem. Each of the over seven thousand funds that now exist is designed to fulfill many different goals, and unsuspecting, inexperienced consumers may find them confusing. At any rate, typical mutual fund literature lists three primary advantages to them:

1. diversification;

2. professional management; and

3. lower expenses.

The mutual funds discussed and listed in this book (see Figures 8.5a and 8.5b) were generally chosen to help you achieve your goals by reducing risk through proper diversification. A portfolio of less than $125,000 would be extremely hard-pressed to become properly diversified without the use of mutual funds, regardless of what some brokers and financial advisors will tell you.

Be extremely wary of the excessive costs involved in strategies that avoid mutual funds in smaller portfolios. I will stress again that most brokers and advisors are paid commissions and often push their individual stocks and bonds to smaller investors so they can enhance their own commissions, rather than addressing the needs of their clients. Brokers and commission-oriented financial planners sell mutual funds which have costs that can be up to four or five times higher than no-load/low-fee funds.

Because of their ability to pool the investment capital from thousands of different investors, mutual funds have a great ability to diversify, which significantly reduces risk. Of course, with billions of dollars under management (upon which to charge fees), most funds have top talent guiding their portfolios. Many of these managers specialize in growth, income, or total return funds, for example, and have several years' experience with the same fund. Other mutual funds, called index funds, are designed to do only as well as the stock market or some sort of investment index (such as the S&P 500 or Bond Index); they generally have very low fees because they are not managed.

As mentioned earlier, mutual funds, even those sold by nice, enlightened, socially conscious brokers and commission-oriented financial planners, usually have much higher costs than no-load/low-fee funds. These high fees are often due to marketing costs that don't benefit the investor. Typically, these

## Figure 8.5a

# Mutual Funds

No more than 10% of your portfolio should be held in any one growth fund; 15% in any one balanced fund; or 20% in any one bond fund. Build your diversified portfolio by choosing (beginning with Group I) from each group of the following list of funds.

## Balanced Funds

### Group 1
| | |
|---|---|
| Columbia Balanced | 800 547-1707 |
| Hotchkiss & Wiley Balanced Income | 800 346-7301 |
| T. Rowe Price Balanced | 800 638-5660 / 800 225-5132 |
| Vanguard/Wellesley Income | 800 662-7447 |
| Berwyn Income | 800 992-6757 |
| Dreyfus Premier Balanced | 800 782-6620 |
| Fidelity Puritan | 800 544-8888 |
| Stein Roe Balanced | 800 338-2550 |
| Pax World Fund | 800 767-1729 |

### Group 2
| | |
|---|---|
| American Century Balanced | 800 345-2021 |
| Eclipse Financial Balanced | 800 872-2710 |
| Greenspring | 800 366-3863 |
| State Farm Balanced | 309 766-2029 |
| Vanguard Asset Allocation | 800 662-7447 |
| Vanguard STAR | 800 662-7447 |
| Fidelity Asset Manager | 800 544-8888 |
| Preferred Asset Allocation | 800 662-4769 |

### Group 3
| | |
|---|---|
| Dodge & Cox Balanced | 800 621-3979 / 415 981-1710 |
| Invesco Total Return | 800 525-8085 |
| Lindner Dividend Investment | 800 995-7777 / 314 727-5305 |
| AHA Balanced | 800 445-1341 |
| CGM Mutual | 800 345-4048 |
| Schwab Asset Balanced Growth | 800 435-4000 |
| Scudder Balanced | 800 SCUDDER |
| Strong Balanced | 800 368-1030 |
| Lindner Dividend Fund | 888 995-7777 |

**Figure 8.5a** *continued*

## Stock Funds

### Group 1

| | |
|---|---|
| Pillar Equity Income | 800 932-7782 |
| Schwab Analytics Fund | 800 435-4000 |
| AARP Growth & Income | 800 322-2282 |
| Babson Value | 800 422-2766 |
| Neuberger & Berman Guard | 800 877-9700 |
| Scudder Growth & Income | 800 SCUDDER |
| T. Rowe Price Equity-Income | 800 638-5660 / 800 225-5132 |
| Vanguard/Windsor II | 800 662-7447 |

### Group 2

| | |
|---|---|
| American Century Benham Income & Growth | 800 345-8765 |
| Fidelity Equity Income | 800 544-8888 |
| Marshal Equity Income | 800 236-8560 |
| Janus | 800 525-8983 |
| Nicholas | 800 551-8043 |
| RSI Retirement Core Equity | 800 772-3615 |
| Sit Mid Cap Growth | 800 332-5580 / 612 334-5888 |
| T. Rowe Price Growth Stock | 800 638-5660 / 800 225-5132 |
| T. Rowe Price International Stock | 800 638-5660 / 800 225-5132 |
| Value Line Income | 800 223-0818 |
| Vanguard International Growth | 800 662-7447 |
| Vanguard/Windsor II | 800 662-7447 |

### Group 3

| | |
|---|---|
| Acorn | 800 922-6769 |
| Lindner Growth Investment | 800 995-7777 |
| Meridian | 800 446-6662 |
| Pennsylvania Mutual | 800 221-4268 |
| Scout Regional | 800 422-2766 |
| Lindner Growth Fund | 800 995-7777 |
| Flex Funds (Total Returns, Utilities) | 800 325-3539 |

**Figure 8.5a** *continued*

## Bond Funds

### Tax-Free Funds for Taxable Accounts

### Group 1

| | |
|---|---|
| AARP Insured Tax-Free General Bond | 800 322-2282 |
| Dreyfus Municipal Bond | 800 782-6620 |
| Scudder Managed Municipal Bonds | 800 SCUDDER |
| Vanguard Municipal Intermediate-Term | 800 662-7447 |
| Vanguard Municipal Short-Term | 800 662-7447 |
| Schwab Intermediate Tax Free | 800 435-4000 |

### Group 2

| | |
|---|---|
| Dreyfus Intermediate Municipal | 800 782-6620 |
| Federated Intermediate Municipal | 800 341-7400 / 800 245-5051 |
| Safeco Municipal Bond No-Load | 800 426-6730 / 800 624-5711 |
| Scudder Medium-Term Tax Free | 800 SCUDDER |
| USAA Tax-Exempt Long-Term | 800 382-8722 |
| Vanguard Municipal Insured Long-Term | 800 662-7447 |
| Vanguard Municipal Long-Term | 800 662-7447 |
| Schwab Long-Term Tax Free | 800 435-4000 |

## International Stock Funds

| | |
|---|---|
| Sogen International (No-Load Version Only) | 800 334-2143 |
| BT Investment International | 800 730-1313 |
| Harbor International | 800 442-1050 |
| Managers International Equity | 800 835-3879 |
| IVY International A | 800 456-5111 |
| Lindner International | 888 995-7777 |
| U.S. Global Leaders Growth | 800 282-2340 |

**Figure 8.5a** *continued*

## Bond Funds

**IRAs, 401ks, Pensions, Charitable Trusts, and Other Tax-Advantaged Vehicles**

### Group 1

| | |
|---|---|
| AARP, GNMA & U.S. Treasury | 800 322-2282 |
| American Century-Benham Short Gov. | 800 345-2021 |
| Columbia Fixed-Income Securities | 800 547-1707 / 503 222-3606 |
| Vanguard Fixed-Income Short-Term Corp. | 800 662-7447 |

### Group 2

| | |
|---|---|
| USAA Income | 800 382-8722 |
| Vanguard Fixed-Income L-T U.S. Treasury | 800 662-7447 |
| Dreyfus Institutional Short-Term Treasury | 800 782-6620 |

### Group 3

| | |
|---|---|
| Pimco Global | 800 800-0952 |
| Brinson Global | 800 448-2430 |
| T. Rowe Price Global Bond | 800 638-5660 / 800 225-5132 |
| Standish International Fixed Income | 800 221-4795 |

## Gold, Natural Resources Funds

### Group 1

| | |
|---|---|
| T. Rowe Price New Era | 800 638-5660 / 800 225-5132 |
| Robertson Stevens Global Natural Resources | 800 766-3863 |

### Group 2

| | |
|---|---|
| Blanchard Precious Metals | 800 829-3863 |
| United Services World Gold | 800 USFUNDS |

## Figure 8.5b

# Social Values Mutual Funds

No more than 10% of your portfolio should be held in any one growth fund; 15% in any one balanced fund; or 20% in any one bond fund. Build your diversified portfolio by choosing (beginning with Group 1) from each group of the following list of funds.

## Growth Funds

### Group 1

| | |
|---|---|
| Aquinas Equity Income | 800 223-7010 |
| Ariel Appreciation | 800 292-7435 |
| *Calvert Fund Strategy | 800 368-2748 |
| *Calvert Social Investment Equity | 800 767-1729 |
| Citizens Index Fund, Institutional | 800 223-7010 |
| Domini Social Equity | 800 762-6814 |
| Green Century Equity Fund | 800 934-7338 |
| MMA Praxis Growth | 800 977-2947 |
| Rightime Social Awareness | 800 242-1421 |

### Group 2

| | |
|---|---|
| Ariel Growth | 800 292-7435 |
| Bridgeway Ultra Small Companies | 800 661-3550 |
| Calvert Capital Accumulation | 800 368-2748 |
| Citizens Emerging | 800 223-7010 |
| Delaware Group Quantum Fund A | 800 523-4640 |
| Dreyfus Third Century | 800 554-4611 |
| Parnassus Fund | 800 999-3505 |

### Group 3

| | |
|---|---|
| American Trust Allegiance | 800 385-7003 |
| Aquinas Equity | 800 423-6369 |
| Bridgeway Socially Responsible | 800 661-3550 |
| *Calvert Managed | 800 368-2748 |
| Citizens Index Fund | 800 223-7010 |
| DEVCAP | 800 371-2855 |
| Hudson Investors Fund | 800 483-7664 |
| Neuberger & Berman | 800 877-9700 |
| New Alternatives | 800 423-8383 |
| Pax World Growth Fund | 800 767-1729 |
| Security Social Awareness Fund | 800 888-2461 |
| Timothy Plan Institutional | 800 846-7526 |
| Citizens, Index Fund, Retail | 800 223-7010 |
| Womens Equity Mutual Fund | 415 547-9135 |

**Figure 8.5b** *continued*

## Balanced Funds

### Group 1
Pax World Fund                          800 767-1729

### Group 2
Calvert Social Investment               800 368-2748
Green Century Balanced                  800 934-7336

### Group 3
Aquinas Balanced                        800 423-6369
Parnassus                               800 999-3505

## Bond Funds

### Group 1
Aquinas Fixed Income Bond               800 423-6369
MMA Praxis Intermediate                 800 977-2947

### Group 2
*Calvert Income                         800 368-2748
Parnassus Fixed Income                  800 999-3505

### Group 3
Citizens Income Fund                    800 223-7010
*Calvert Social Bond                    800 368-2748

### Group 4
Eclipse Ultra Short Term                800 872-2710

## International Stock Funds

*Calvert World Value Intl. Equity       800 368-2748
Citizens Global Equity                  800 223-7010

**Figure 8.5b** *continued*

## Gold and Natural Resource Funds

| | |
|---|---|
| T. Rowe Price New Era | 800 638-5660 |
| Blanchard Precious Metals | 800 829-3863 |
| United Services World Gold | 800 USFUNDS |

## Unique Funds

| | |
|---|---|
| Amana Islamic Growth Fund (Growth) | 800 728-8762 |
| Amana Islamic Income Fund (Bond) | 800 728-8762 |
| America Asia Allocation Growth | 703 356-3720 |
| *Calvert New Africa (Growth) | 800 368-2748 |
| Cruelty Free Value | 800 662-9992 |
| Meyers Pride Value | 800 410-3337 |
| Total Return Utilities Fund | 800 325-3539 |
| Utilities Growth Fund | 800 325-3539 |
| Womens Equity Mutual Fund (Growth) | 415 547-9135 |

For your personal Cash Management account, consider the following two funds:

| | |
|---|---|
| Calvert Social Money Market | 800 368-2748 |
| Citizens Working Assets Money Fund | 800 223-7010 |

• Calvert funds are load funds, though some brokerage firms allow you to buy the funds no-load. Make sure you do not pay a load on Calvert funds.

Source: Lipper Analytical Services

fees are charged as a front-end fee, up to 8.5 percent ($850 on a $10,000 investment), or they might catch you with back-end surrender fees, which serve as deferred sales charges. Funds that use these deferred/back-end loads/back-end fees (whatever you prefer to call them) overcharge you on an annual basis in order to pay about 4 percent commission to their sales-people. Using funds with expensive front or back loads is unnecessary; similarly, equally viable funds (without such costs) are available. All of the funds listed in Figure 8.5 control their expenses and usually have fees that are significantly lower than those charged by their loaded counterparts.

Unfortunately, many financial institutions and financial planners are dumb-ing down their services by using mutual funds exclusively to build client portfolios. Some firms charge up to 3 percent annually (if you add up the hidden mutual fund fees). Simply stated, you don't need to pay an advisor big fees to select your mutual funds: do it yourself.

Realize that all mutual funds have fees and expenses. If you like the idea of someone doing your mutual fund portfolio for you, pay them a flat fee a year or a very modest fee (under 4/10 of 1 percent) based on the size of your portfolio for the peace of mind you might receive.

Don't, under any circumstances, use a commissioned person to select any investments for you. Unless they are fee-only and experienced, don't use them. And beyond their fee schedule, your portfolio manager should be buying individual stocks and bonds, not just mutual funds. If they mainly use open-ended mutual funds, your portfolio is most likely being dumbed down to mediocre returns and excessive fees by a manager who is basically providing you with bookkeeping services.

You shouldn't, of course, choose a fund simply because it has lower fees. By going directly to the mutual fund companies or using an investment manager, you can avoid paying high marketing fees to brokers and other commissioned professionals. Several funds specialize in working with money managers and educated investors who prefer going direct. Fund groups such as Vanguard, T. Rowe Price, Scudder, Stevens & Clark, SEI, Pimco, Schwab, Federated, Citizens, and TIAA/CREF all have designed their products for individuals and professionals who make their decisions based on merit and careful analysis rather than the pressure tactics used by brokers. Also, be aware that a few so-called no-load funds have loads on some of their portfolios.

Some load mutual funds have excellent management and a history of solid returns, to be sure. And if you presently own a load fund, it may make sense to keep it since you have already paid the front-end fee. Some of my favorite load funds for transfer are Templeton, MFS, Sogen, Putnam, Franklin, American Funds, Calvert, and Fidelity.

When switching funds from balanced or stock funds in your taxable do-it-yourself portfolio, always switch the fund with the smallest capital gain. Also, for taxable accounts, try to wait twelve months before you switch in order to lower your tax liability (don't wait unless you are only a few months from a switch). If you have held a mutual fund for at least twelve months, the capital gain rate is only 20 percent. Tax-smart principles apply when switching the equity or balanced holdings of your tax-favored IRA, retirement, or pension accounts. For example, if you need to move $50,000 from stocks, and have sufficient funds to move it all from your IRA, do it from the tax-favored account (instead of a taxable account) to save taxes. You don't need to adjust each portfolio identically. Tax-smart asset allocation is the key.

I often interview mutual fund managers to decipher exactly what their goals are. Who do they see as their customer? Is it the young, aggressive hotshot who wants quick returns, or the retired person investing for an ever-increasing income and capital pool? Do they have any of their own money (How much?) in the fund they are managing? Knowing details of how a fund manager operates allows me to feel comfortable in recommending the fund to clients. Obviously, this is difficult to do on your own, but be sure to read the prospectus, Web site marketing literature, Lipper Reports, or Morningstar Reports of a fund to understand their goals and philosophies.

Mutual funds allow you to purchase and sell shares at the day's-end share price. They are very easy to sell and are usually sold without cost (although some have back-end fees, as mentioned earlier, to be avoided if possible). If you choose to purchase mutual fund shares through a discount broker, be prepared for the modest fee they will charge. It's debatable whether this fee is worth it, but the convenience of having your account held at a discount brokerage, with the monthly statements they produce (which eases record-keeping), outweighs the small cost. Many discount brokers offer no-transaction-fee (NTF) funds that allow them to sell you the fund without the small transaction fee. These NTF funds can work well for smaller portfolios but tend to be expensive for larger portfolios. Figure 8.6 lists major discount brokers and summarizes their services and fees.

## Figure 8.6

# Discount Brokers

The sheer number of discount brokers, and the breadth of services they provide, has increased dramatically due to online and other forms of "brokerless" trading. Each excels in certain areas, and while this is a fairly extensive compilation, there are dozens not listed. **Commissions charged and minimum fees change often due to the competitive nature of the industry. Call to verify, as figures listed below could have changed.**

| | Charles Schwab<br>800 435-4000<br>.schwab.com | Fidelity<br>800 544-8666<br>.fidelity.com | Jack White<br>800 233-3411<br>.jackwhiteco.com | Vanguard<br>800 992-8327<br>.vanguard.com |
|---|---|---|---|---|
| Online trading | Yes | Yes | Yes | Yes |
| View account online | Yes | Yes | Yes | Yes |
| Number of no transaction fee mutual funds | Over 825 | Over 700 | Over 1,300 | 0 |
| Minimum transaction fee per trade | ($29.95 online)<br>$39 | ($30.00 online)<br>$38 | ($25 online)<br>$33 | $36.25 |
| Fee per $10,000 mutual fund transaction | .7% of principle | Unavailable | $33 | $35 |
| Annual cost for IRA/less than $5,000 balance | $29 | $24 | $35 | 0 |
| 24-hour trading | Yes | Yes | Yes | Yes |
| Live broker hours | 24 hours/7days | 24 hours/7days | 24 hours/7days | 8–5:30 M–F |
| SIPC and excess insurance to what amount | $99 million | $100 million | $50 million | $25 million |
| Cash management account–checkbook, Visa/MC, cost | Checkbook<br>Visa/MC free | Checkbook<br>Visa/MC free | Checkbook<br>Visa/MC free | Checkbook |
| CMA minimum balance | $2,500 | $10,000 | $3,000 | 0 |

**Figure 8.6** *continued*

| | Muriel Siebert<br>800 872-0711<br>.siebertnet.com | E*Trade<br>800 786-2575<br>.etrade.com. | National<br>Discount Brokers<br>800 888-3999<br>.ndb.com |
|---|---|---|---|
| Online trading | Yes | Yes | Yes |
| View account online | Yes | Yes | Yes |
| Number of no transaction fee mutual funds | Over 600 | 1,100 | Over 500 |
| Minimum transaction fee per trade | ($14.95 online)<br>$37.50 | $14.95 | ($14.95 online)<br>$25 |
| Fee per $10,000 mutual fund transaction | $69.50 | $25 | $20 |
| Annual cost for IRA/less than $5,000 balance | $30 | 0 | $35 |
| 24-hour trading | Yes | Yes | Yes |
| Live broker hours | 7:30–7:30 M–F | 5 AM-6 PM | 7:30–830 M–F |
| SIPC and excess insurance to what amount | $100 million | $50 million | $75 million |
| Cash management account–checkbook, Visa/MC, cost | Checkbook $0<br>Visa/MC $60 | Checkbook | Checkbook<br>Visa/MC |
| CMA minimum balance | 0 | $1,000 | 0/$10,000 |

## Figure 8.6 *continued*

| | AmericanExpress Financial Direct 800 297-7010 .american express.com | Ameritrade 800 669-3900 .ameritrade.com | DLJ Direct 800 825-5723 .dljdirect.com |
|---|---|---|---|
| Online trading | Yes | Yes | Yes |
| View account online | Yes | Yes | Yes |
| Number of no transaction fee mutual funds | Over 200 | 0 | 600 |
| Minimum transaction fee per trade | ($24.95 online) $49 | ($8 online) $18 | $20 |
| Fee per $10,000 mutual fund transaction | 0 for recordkeeping, $40 for early redemption | $18 | $35 |
| Annual cost for IRA/less than $5,000 balance | $29 | 0 | $35 |
| 24-hour trading | Yes | Yes | Yes |
| Live broker hours | 7–12 M–F, 9–6 S–S | 6–10 M–F | 7–1AM M–F |
| SIPC and excess insurance to what amount | $25 million | $10.5 million | $50 million |
| Cash management account–checkbook, Visa/MC, cost | Checkbook Visa/MC | No | Checkbook Visa/MC |
| CMA minimum balance | 0 | $2,000 | 0 |

# chapter nine

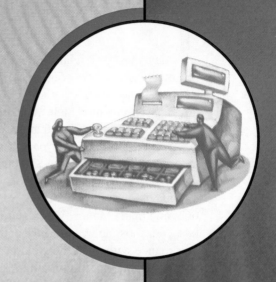

# Dollar-Cost-Averaging

Today, most physicians have access to money purchase types of retirement plans where consistent monthly deposits can be made. 401ks and tax-sheltered 403(b) plans (TSAs) are two of the most common self-directed retirement vehicles, allowing individuals the flexibility to make allocation decisions. This feature also suits them well for dollar-cost-averaging, a simple do-it-yourself strategy that is an effective way to make monthly deposits of $10 to $10,000 into select no-load mutual funds.

The magic of dollar-cost-averaging is simply a matter of time, diversification, and mathematics. When starting out, the idea is to make payments into your most aggressive investments, and then rebalance quarterly in accordance with what the yield is on stocks. This approach should be kept up until you acquire approximately $10,000 through the use of balanced or asset allocation mutual funds from the list provided in chapter eight. As you can see in Figure 9.1 (Dollar-Cost-Averaging), dollar-cost-averaging won't guarantee you success in a falling market on a short-term basis. But markets trend up over extended periods, and the upside of investing into a falling market is that you are buying more shares with each investment.

Along with the individual features and restrictions of your retirement plan, the following rules should be adhered to:

1. If you are only allowed to rebalance quarterly, check the stock yield ten days before you are able to switch. If yields suggest a change, do it then.

2. If you are allowed unlimited rebalancing options and are making consistent deposits, try to rebalance at least quarterly. Otherwise, do so on yield changes.

3. Use managed funds. Avoid indexed funds, if possible.

4. If gold/natural resource funds are unavailable, substitute international and/or stock funds. If no stock funds, use balanced funds. If no balanced funds, substitute 50 percent stock/50 percent bond funds.

More and more physicians are becoming eligible to take advantage of tax-sheltered annuities/403(b) because they are prevalent in hospitals and educational institutions. Often, they are the only retirement plan available in these physician workplaces. The maximum yearly amount that can be funded into a TSA is $30,000, of which only $9,500 can be contributed by the physician participant. The balance must come from the employer.

| Figure 9.1 |
| --- |

# Dollar-Cost-Averaging
**($100 /month = $400 total)**

| Market | Sideways | | Rising | | Falling | |
| --- | --- | --- | --- | --- | --- | --- |
| | Stock Price | Number of Shares | Stock Price | Number of Shares | Stock Price | Number of Shares |
| 1st month | $10 | 10 | $10 | 10 | $10 | 10 |
| 2nd month | 9 | 11 | 14 | 7 | 7 | 14 |
| 3rd month | 11 | 9 | 20 | 5 | 5 | 20 |
| 4th month | 11 | 9 | 25 | 4 | 4 | 25 |
| **Total shares** | | **39** | | **26** | | **69** |

$$39 \times \$11 = \$429$$
$$-\$400$$
$$\$\ 29 \text{ gain}$$

$$26 \times \$25 = \$650$$
$$-\$400$$
$$\$250 \text{ gain}$$

$$69 \times \$4 = \$276$$
$$-\$400$$
$$\$124 \text{ loss}$$

# Make Dollar-Cost-Averaging Work

- *Make a commitment:* To reap the rewards of the compounding phenomenon, discipline yourself to set aside a certain amount monthly. Money and time work magic together; start early.
- *Determine your willingness to take risks:* Aggressive, growth, balanced, yield, or capital preservation.

- *Follow the yield:* You can find listings for the current dividend yields on both the Dow Jones and S&P 500 in such business publications as *The Wall Street Journal, Barron's*, and *Investors Business Daily.*
- *Identify your investor type:* Decide on an appropriate investment program based on your risk tolerance.

TIAA/CREF is the most common TSA provider at hospitals and universities. They have fine products that are well priced and ideally suited for dollar-cost-averaging. Once your account reaches sufficient size ($10,000 or so), however, you should move it into a do-it-yourself strategy.

New money in a recently created TSA should be aggressively invested favoring growth and international funds, even if the stock market is significantly overvalued and if your annual contributions are less than 25 percent of your portfolio value. Thus, once your portfolio is over four times your annual deposit, you should manage it under the do-it-yourself strategy, although the new money should still be aggressively invested to take full advantage of dollar-cost-averaging. Other great TSA products are available through no-load mutual fund groups like Vanguard, Calvert, Citizens, etc. Vanguard's phone number is 800 992-8327, and TIAA/CREF's is 800 842-2776.

# Dollar-Cost-Averaging Sample Portfolios

Use the five examples shown in Figures 9.2–9.6 as a template to structure your own monthly payments into an investment portfolio. As mentioned earlier, when beginning this strategy (before you have amassed $10,000), make your payments into your most aggressive investments. Investors who manage portfolios of any size can factor in their risk tolerance and take advantage of the dollar-cost-averaging strategy. Simply identify which type of investor you are (aggressive, growth, balanced, yield, or capital preservation), and use the examples to begin your savings program.

## Figure 9.2

# Aggressive Investor

### 3% Yield

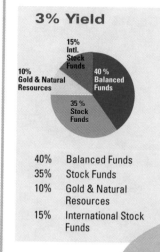

15% Intl. Stock Funds
10% Gold & Natural Resources
40% Balanced Funds
35% Stock Funds

40%    Balanced Funds
35%    Stock Funds
10%    Gold & Natural
       Resources
15%    International Stock
       Funds

### 4% Yield

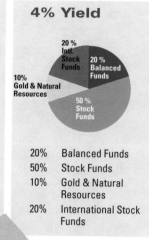

20% Intl. Stock Funds
20% Balanced Funds
10% Gold & Natural Resources
50% Stock Funds

20%    Balanced Funds
50%    Stock Funds
10%    Gold & Natural
       Resources
20%    International Stock
       Funds

### 5% Yield

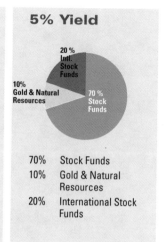

20% Intl. Stock Funds
10% Gold & Natural Resources
70% Stock Funds

70%    Stock Funds
10%    Gold & Natural
       Resources
20%    International Stock
       Funds

### Example:

Dr A is an **aggressive** investor with $400 per month to invest. He looks up the yield and it is **4%**. He divides his monthly allotment like this:

(20% of $400)  **$ 80**    into a balanced fund (ie, _____).

(50% of $400)  **$200**    into stock funds. He further divvies these into two stock funds:
                           (ie, $100 _____)
                           (ie, $100 _____).

(20% of $400)  **$ 80**    into an international stock fund
                           (ie, _____).

(10% of $400)  **$ 40**    into a gold and natural resource fund
                           (ie, _____).

**Figure 9.3**

# Growth Investor

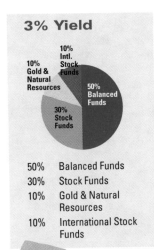

### 3% Yield

10% Intl. Stock Funds
10% Gold & Natural Resources
50% Balanced Funds
30% Stock Funds

| 50% | Balanced Funds |
| 30% | Stock Funds |
| 10% | Gold & Natural Resources |
| 10% | International Stock Funds |

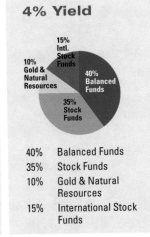

### 4% Yield

15% Intl. Stock Funds
10% Gold & Natural Resources
40% Balanced Funds
35% Stock Funds

| 40% | Balanced Funds |
| 35% | Stock Funds |
| 10% | Gold & Natural Resources |
| 15% | International Stock Funds |

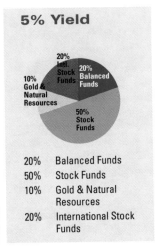

### 5% Yield

20% Intl. Stock Funds
20% Balanced Funds
10% Gold & Natural Resources
50% Stock Funds

| 20% | Balanced Funds |
| 50% | Stock Funds |
| 10% | Gold & Natural Resources |
| 20% | International Stock Funds |

### Example:

Dr G is a **growth** investor with $500 per month to invest. She looks up the yield and it is **3%**. She divides her monthly allotment like this:

(50% of $500) **$250** into a balanced fund. She further divvies these into two balanced funds
(ie, $125 _____)
(ie, $125 _____).

(30% of $500) **$150** into stock funds. She further divvies these into two stock funds
(ie, $75 _____)
(ie, $75 _____).

(10% of $500) **$ 50** into a gold and natural resources fund
(ie, _____).

(10% of $500) **$ 50** into an international fund
(ie, _____).

**Figure 9.4**

# Balanced Investor

## 3% Yield

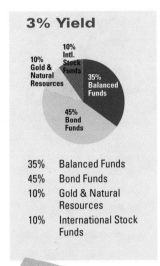

| | |
|---|---|
| 35% | Balanced Funds |
| 45% | Bond Funds |
| 10% | Gold & Natural Resources |
| 10% | International Stock Funds |

## 4% Yield

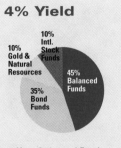

| | |
|---|---|
| 45% | Balanced Funds |
| 35% | Bond Funds |
| 10% | Gold & Natural Resources |
| 10% | International Stock Funds |

## 5% Yield

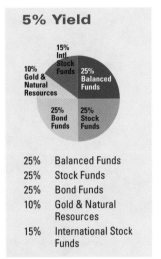

| | |
|---|---|
| 25% | Balanced Funds |
| 25% | Stock Funds |
| 25% | Bond Funds |
| 10% | Gold & Natural Resources |
| 15% | International Stock Funds |

### Example:

Dr B is a **balanced** investor with $300 per month to invest. He looks up the yield and it is **3%**. He divides his monthly allotment like this:

(35% of $300) **$105** into a balanced fund (ie, _____).

(45% of $300) **$135** into bond funds. He further divvies these into two bond funds:
(ie, $50 _____)
(ie, $85 _____).

(10% of $300) **$ 30** into a gold and natural resources fund (ie, _____).

(10% of $300) **$ 30** into an international stock fund (ie, _____).

## Figure 9.5

# Yield Investor

### 3% Yield

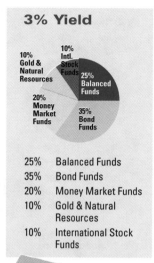

10% Gold & Natural Resources
10% Intl. Stock Funds
25% Balanced Funds
20% Money Market Funds
35% Bond Funds

| 25% | Balanced Funds |
| 35% | Bond Funds |
| 20% | Money Market Funds |
| 10% | Gold & Natural Resources |
| 10% | International Stock Funds |

### 4% Yield

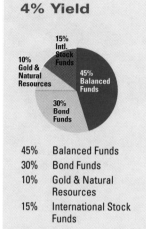

15% Intl. Stock Funds
10% Gold & Natural Resources
45% Balanced Funds
30% Bond Funds

| 45% | Balanced Funds |
| 30% | Bond Funds |
| 10% | Gold & Natural Resources |
| 15% | International Stock Funds |

### 5% Yield

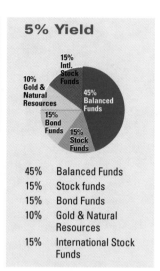

15% Intl. Stock Funds
10% Gold & Natural Resources
45% Balanced Funds
15% Bond Funds
15% Stock Funds

| 45% | Balanced Funds |
| 15% | Stock funds |
| 15% | Bond Funds |
| 10% | Gold & Natural Resources |
| 15% | International Stock Funds |

### Example:

Dr Y is a **yield** investor with $300 per month to invest. She looks up the yield and it is **3%**. She divides her monthly allotment like this:

(25% of $300) **$ 75** into a balanced fund (ie, _____).

(35% of $300) **$105** into bond funds. She further divvies these into two bond funds:
(ie, $50 _____)
(ie, $55 _____).

(20% of $300) **$ 60** into a money market fund (ie, _____).

(10% of $300) **$ 30** into a gold and natural resources fund (ie, _____).

(10% of $300) **$ 30** into an international stock fund (ie, _____).

## Figure 9.6

# Capital Preservation Investor

### 3% Yield

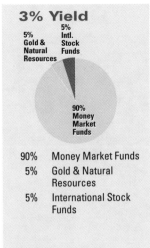

5% Gold & Natural Resources

5% Intl. Stock Funds

90% Money Market Funds

| | |
|---|---|
| 90% | Money Market Funds |
| 5% | Gold & Natural Resources |
| 5% | International Stock Funds |

### 4% Yield

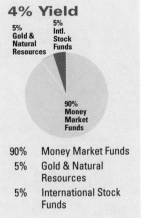

5% Gold & Natural Resources

5% Intl. Stock Funds

90% Money Market Funds

| | |
|---|---|
| 90% | Money Market Funds |
| 5% | Gold & Natural Resources |
| 5% | International Stock Funds |

### 5% Yield

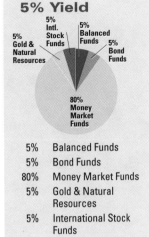

5% Intl. Stock Funds

5% Balanced Funds

5% Gold & Natural Resources

5% Bond Funds

80% Money Market Funds

| | |
|---|---|
| 5% | Balanced Funds |
| 5% | Bond Funds |
| 80% | Money Market Funds |
| 5% | Gold & Natural Resources |
| 5% | International Stock Funds |

### Example:

Dr Y is a **capital preservation** investor with $300 per month to invest. She looks up the yield and it is **3%**. She divides her monthly allotment like this:

(90% of $300) **$270** into a money market fund (ie, _____).

(5% of $300) **$ 15** into a gold and natural resources fund (ie, _____).

(5% of $300) **$ 15** into an international stock fund (ie, _____).

# chapter ten

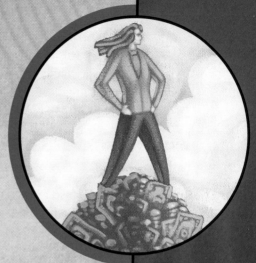

# Once Retired, Plan to Live Forever

As discussed in chapter seven, your investment portfolio needs to be managed competently and wisely; but unlike when you retire, your money continues to work. In fact, in retirement your money's job becomes much more demanding and important. No matter how well your portfolio grew throughout your working life, though, you need to take a completely objective look at how it needs to perform in retirement.

In other chapters, we discussed using cycles to help avoid investing into market manias. We also learned how to identify investment opportunities by monitoring the dividend yield paid on the stock market to tell us whether stocks were to be avoided or embraced. I am a very big fan of retirement portfolios that are designed to capitalize on income that is earned from an emphasis on dividends and interest-oriented equity investments. A good retirement portfolio goal is to have interest income equal to at least 80 percent of your income withdrawal needs. To accomplish this, search for equities (stocks, both domestic and foreign) where a significant part of the return comes from predictable income dividends. Energy utility stocks, real estate investment trusts, and stocks of companies that are unpopular (not unpromising) can help beef up the income of portfolios. In addition, we favor income-oriented convertible bonds (bonds that can be exchanged for stocks) and convertible preferred stocks with favorable dividends, either individually or in closed-end or open-end mutual funds.

If you use the do-it-yourself strategy outlined in chapter eight, emphasis should be placed on equity income and convertible bond mutual funds. In Figure 10.1 (Your Money Doesn't Retire), we illustrate how a bear market might affect your portfolio, using a strategy similar to the do-it-yourself strategy. Notice that the income from the portfolio does not go down, even though the portfolio value goes down. This is because company managements are forward-looking with their dividend policies, realize the economy is cyclical, anticipate that there will be periods of slow or no economic growth, and stay disciplined through normal business cycles. In most cases, companies that pay good dividends (energy utilities, telecommunications, real estate leasing, etc) are usually businesses that are only modestly affected by economic cycles. The other way you can buy great companies that pay hefty dividends is to wait for a bear market to decrease the price of the company stock to the point where the dividend has the potential to become a significant part of the investment's total return.

Over the history of the stock market, approximately half of all returns have come from cash dividends. This is why one of the main thrusts of the do-it-yourself strategy is to buy stocks aggressively when the average yield is

**Figure 10.1**

# Your Money Doesn't Retire

## Aggressive Retiree ± 35%—Hits Bear Market

|  | Year 1 | Year 2 | Year 3 | Year 4 | Year 5 |
|---|---|---|---|---|---|
| Portfolio beginning of year | $1,000,000 | $1,010,000 | $800,000 | $750,000 | $640,000 |
| Net income for year | 50,000 | 50,000 | 50,000 | 50,000 | 50,000 |
| Income withdrawal for year | 60,000 | 60,000 | 60,000 | 60,000 | 60,000 |
| Portfolio end of year | $1,010,000 | $ 800,000 | $750,000 | $640,000 | $740,000 |

## Balanced Retiree ± 25%—Hits Bear Market

|  | Year 1 | Year 2 | Year 3 | Year 4 | Year 5 |
|---|---|---|---|---|---|
| Portfolio beginning of year | $1,000,000 | $1,008,000 | $900,000 | $800,000 | $750,000 |
| Net income for year | 50,000 | 50,000 | 50,000 | 50,000 | 50,000 |
| Income withdrawal for year | 54,000 | 54,000 | 54,000 | 54,000 | 54,000 |
| Portfolio end of year | $1,008,000 | $ 900,000 | $800,000 | $750,000 | $835,000 |

## Yield Investor ± 15%—Hits Bear Market

|  | Year 1 | Year 2 | Year 3 | Year 4 | Year 5 |
|---|---|---|---|---|---|
| Portfolio beginning of year | $1,000,000 | $1,002,000 | $900,000 | $875,000 | $850,000 |
| Net income for year | 55,000 | 55,000 | 55,000 | 55,000 | 55,000 |
| Income withdrawal for year | 48,000 | 48,000 | 48,000 | 48,000 | 48,000 |
| Portfolio end of year | $1,002,000 | $ 900,000 | $875,000 | $850,000 | $900,000 |

*Note:* The above is for illustration only and is to show how a bear market might affect a do-it-yourself portfolio if it became very severe. Understand that with any investment strategy, there are no guarantees.

5 percent or so. That 5 percent amounts to half the historical 10 percent average return of stocks over time.

To balance out your portfolio of securities, income investments will be used, that is, fixed preferred stocks, corporate bonds, government bonds, and other fixed-income–oriented investments, purchased either through a mutual fund or by an individual portfolio manager. Fixed-income securities range from the most conservative Treasury bill to the most aggressive junk bond or junk-rated preferred stock. It is usually best to be extremely diversified with your portfolio—even the income portion. If you use mutual funds, take comfort in knowing that they have built-in diversification.

I have found that many investors are lazy when it comes to managing the income portion of their portfolio. The tendency is to buy and forget. The cyclical nature of interest rates creates opportunities in the bond market, and over time bonds fall in and out of favor due to their industry, maturity, put or call provisions, ratings, liquidity constraints, etc. This volatility is quite often hard to decipher, but extra returns can be earned without adding extra risk just by being aware and willing to take the chance to sell overvalued or buy undervalued fixed-income investments. Depending on your risk constraints, when the dividend yields are high on stocks, there is often an opportunity to buy corporate bonds at great prices. During periods where dividend yields are low, it is logical to emphasize good, safe, predictable US Government bond funds in your portfolio. Also, be ready to switch into corporate bond–oriented funds when you move more aggressively into stock and balanced funds with your do-it-yourself portfolio.

> **The average fee-only financial advisor serving physicians found that . . .**
> Their average retired client's income is between $75,000 and $220,000 annually.

# The Speed Limit

Some rules of thumb to follow with your income-providing retirement portfolio are as follows:

1. Try to have your portfolio straight income/dividend yields equal to at least 80 percent of your retirement income needs.

2. Stay very diversified; never invest more than 2.5 percent of your portfolio in any one individual common stock or bond unless it's a US Government bond or a diversified mutual fund.

3. Always use discount brokers who are fully insured to the total value of your portfolio through the Securities Investors Protection Corporation (SIPC), as well as excess insurance through another well-rated company.

4. Have an investment philosophy to guide your portfolio, such as the one offered in chapter seven, or a philosophy based on the do-it-yourself strategy.

5. Have your portfolio reviewed by an objective professional every year or so if you're doing-it-yourself and every few years if you use a fee-only registered investment advisor, just to make sure all is well.

6. Review mutual funds at least monthly if you manage your own portfolio, and review individual stocks and bonds daily (should you buy more, sell, or hold) on the Internet or via another news source.

7. Do not fall in love with any one security—stay objective with your investments because they are the tools to ensure you have income security.

8. Don't make dramatic changes in your portfolio; make changes slowly as cycles change, and don't allow anyone to rattle you into making changes unless they seem logical and consistent with your goals. When in doubt, get a second opinion.

9. Be realistic. The stock market has returned only 10 percent per year on average for its history until recently, when the outrageous mania with large stocks upped the average to 12 percent. History shows that the stock market will be nudged back to reasonableness by a spontaneous event like a bear market or just by going sideways for a long time, providing low returns.

10. No matter what, don't draw over 6 percent income on your retirement portfolio (except for brief periods); 3 percent to 5 percent is better, depending on your risk tolerance, needs, and portfolio constraints.

11. Think globally; your portfolio should reflect a global perspective, and the mutual funds or individual securities you choose should have a global bias.

12. In retirement, remember that if your portfolio doubles, it won't change your lifestyle; but if it drops in half, it surely will.

# Don't Worry, Be Happy

If your portfolio ever causes you to lose sleep, you need to change something. If you lose sleep because its value fluctuates too much, then reduce risk, even if that means reducing your income. Often, anxiety over your investment portfolio is simply caused by a lack of understanding. Sometimes the best thing to do when your portfolio causes you undue stress is to review each security in it. You should ask, "Would I buy this security today?" as you review each security. One of our favorite sayings in regard to securities is "when in doubt, throw it out"; a legitimate time to worry is when you start "hoping" an investment will perform better because you have certainly lost your objectivity. If you can't do-it-yourself and relax, then hire somebody that you trust.

# Hiring Professionals

Choosing an investment professional to help you manage your portfolio can be a trying, time-consuming task, but it is a very important one and well worth the effort expended. Your mission is to find someone you feel absolutely comfortable with, someone who has a firm structured to ensure long-term excellence in money management. As discussed in other chapters, whoever you hire should be a fee-only (all the time) manager, not fees plus occasional commissions or any other configuration. In order to stay completely objective, a money manager simply cannot be influenced by commissions. Brokerage firms use commissioned salespeople to sell you stuff. In addition, it's best to only hire professionals with at least ten years of discretionary investment management experience. And then, with a legal pad in hand and this book in front of you, ask a potential manager the questions listed in Figure 10.2.

It's your job during this meeting to listen very attentively. If the person you are chatting with is a marketing person for the firm, set up a conference call with the specific person who will manage your portfolio. I am face-to-face oriented; if necessary, I would suggest flying to see the individual manager who will make your investment decisions. Your money and retirement security are worth this extra effort.

Whoever makes the decisions on your portfolio should hold an MBA or have the equivalent experience with financial markets over a significant amount of time. They should also have excellent backup professionals, hopefully some younger ones who will be able to serve your needs when the senior people retire. I am also partial to smaller investment management firms because this allows for entrepreneurial enthusiasm and the ability to look at each client as an important and valuable piece of the firm.

---

**Figure 10.2**

# Tough Questions to Ask a Potential Portfolio Manager

1. Describe your average client.
2. How long have you been in business? How long in this specialized or specific area?
3. How many other physician clients do you have?
4. Do you have any one client who represents more than 10 percent of your income in the last twelve months?
5. Do you plan on staying in this profession? How long?
6. Do you really love the investment business?
7. What business/professional associations do you belong to?
8. Can you give me two professional references to call regarding your character?
9. Can you give me two clients to call as references (clients for at least three years)?
10. How do you get most of your business—referrals, advertising, buying another practice, etc?
11. Who is your ideal client?
12. What determines your pricing, and is your fee negotiable?
13. How much of my portfolio management work will you do, and how much will an associate of yours do?
14. Have you ever declared bankruptcy?
15. What are your business goals?
16. Do I have access to all documents in your file about my specific situation?
17. What assurances do I have of complete confidentiality?
18. How long has your staff been with you?
19. Do you like your job?
20. Have you ever been treated for alcoholism or drug abuse, or been in jail?
21. Who backs you up?
22. Who will have custody of my assets?
23. Are you growth oriented, value oriented, or a balanced manager?
24. Do you specialize in one type of management?
25. Are you appropriate to manage all of my money, or are you a specialty manager?
26. What has portfolio performance been?
27. How do you keep up on investments in my portfolio?
28. Do you consider taxes when buying and selling investments?
29. Where do you get your investment ideas?
30. Can I see your company's written investment philosophy?
31. Can I see an actual portfolio?
32. Does your firm's investment philosophy include social screening?
33. I realize you are fee-only all the time. Why is this, and is there a benefit to me if my advisor collects commissions as well?
34. What makes you better than the people down the street?

## Cruise Lines

| | | |
|---|---|---|
| American Canadian Caribbean Line | 800 556-7450 | www.accl-smallships.com |
| American Hawaii Cruises | 800 765-7450 | www.cruisehawaii.com |
| Carnival Cruise Lines | 800 327-9501 | www.carnival.com |
| Celebrity Cruises | 800 437-3111 | www.celebritycruises.com |
| Clipper Cruise Line | 800 325-0010 | www.clippercruise.com |
| Costa Cruises | 800 462-6782 | www.costacruises.com/home.html |
| Crystal Cruises | 800 446-6620 | www.crystalcruises.com |
| Cunard Line | 800 528-6273 | www.cunardline.com |
| Delta Queen Steamboat Co | 800 458-6789 | www.deltaqueen.com |
| Discovery Cruises | 800 937-4477 | www.discoverycruises.com |
| Fantasy Cruises & Tours | 800 798-7722 | www.fantasycruises.com |
| Holland America | 800 426-0327 | www.hollandamerica.com |
| Norwegian Cruise Line | 800 327-7030 | www.ncl.com |
| Premier Cruises | 800 327-7113 | www.premiercruises.com |
| Princess Cruises | 800 421-0522 | www.princesscruises.com |
| Renaissance Cruises | 800 525-5350 | www.renaissancecruises.com |
| Royal Caribbean International | 800 327-6700 | www.rccl.com |
| Royal Olympic Cruises | 800 221-2470 | www.epirotiki.com |
| Seabourn Cruise Line | 800 929-9595 | www.seabourn.com |
| Windjammer Barefoot | 800 327-2601 | www.windjammer.com |
| Windstar Cruises | 800 258-7245 | www.windstarcruises.com |
| World Explorer Cruises | 800 854-3835 | www.wecruise.com |

Your portfolio must be managed like you'll live forever. You absolutely can't assume a specific year you expect to die. Look at your portfolio as if it were a chicken that lays eggs. You wouldn't want to eat the chicken, (ie, principle). Nor do you want to eat all of the eggs (ie, return) because you will want to hatch a few (ie, reinvest them) so that you can increase your income to offset inflation.

If you need to increase your investment withdrawal beyond 6 percent per year, consider a fixed joint and 100 percent to your survivor annuity from an insurance company. A fixed annuity will provide you and your spouse with a fixed income you cannot outlive, guaranteed!

The downside with annuities is that you'll forgo inflation protection. Once you and your spouse are dead, the money will stop. But if you reach the point where you need more income, don't draw down your principal; buy a fixed annuity from highly rated companies with the help of a fee-only advisor. Also, diversify your annuity income by choosing three to five different annuity companies, just in case.

**The average fee-only financial advisor serving physicians found that . . .**
Their average retired client is drawing 3.5 percent to 8.5 percent from their retirement plan and reinvesting their excess earnings.

# chapter eleven

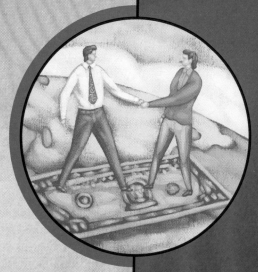

# Monitor Your Progress: Straight Talk on Growing Old

**A**ll aspects of your finances should be reviewed periodically to keep up with the various situational changes in your life. For example, your insurance needs will change dramatically as your net worth increases and your liabilities decrease (children grow older, etc). And because insurance is a costly and extremely important component of any financial plan, it needs to be reviewed at least annually, first, to make sure you're not wasting money on unnecessary coverage, and second, to make sure you're appropriately covered.

Your tax situation will change many times throughout your life, and this is where a good, advice-oriented CPA or tax-oriented financial professional can earn their keep. Also, your goals and lifestyle needs will change, which will affect your financial plan and may require adjustments to your will or trusts. It's a healthy discipline to review your budget annually in order to make sure you're being efficient and conscious of where your money is going. In addition, you should check the interest rates on all of your debt obligations annually to make sure that you're not wasting money unnecessarily.

Perhaps the most important financial entity you should review periodically is the progress of your portfolio. Net worth that turns into income-producing investments is the key to any retirement plan. Nothing is more important than building net worth prudently and effectively through the management of your retirement plan portfolio(s). The stock market fluctuates, bonds have cyclical influences, interest rates change, and money market investments don't do much at all except preserve (not grow) capital. There will be low times over the life of your portfolio, when you will wonder why you ever chose a strategy that emphasized stocks and equities. But if you choose a strategy that emphasizes bonds and money market investments, there will be times when you look at your meager return and say, "If I had only invested in stocks, I would've made a killing and probably could retire today." No investment is perfect for any period, be it a month, a year, a decade, or a lifetime. Don't believe anyone who says differently.

# Manage Your Portfolio to Win All the Time

Over time, the only proven investment winner is not a specific investment but rather a management strategy designed to win no matter what, one that recognizes the cyclical nature of investment markets and realizes that certain investments (like stocks ) will become highly overvalued due to manias.

After the crash of 1929, it took until 1954 for stocks to return to their pre-Depression values. US stock investors who lived through the oil crisis/inflation-induced stock market troubles of the early 1970s waited seventeen years before their portfolios got even with Treasury bills. You simply must stick to a long-term investment strategy that is responsive to an ever-changing world because every type of investment will most certainly have down cycles: gold, collectibles, farmland, oil, stocks, the list goes on; each was touted as the perfect investment at different periods in our history.

As is the case with so many of life's uncertainties, investors often wish to oversimplify their investment strategy. Currently, the dumb-down rage involves asset allocation with a buy-and-hold-forever bias. Investors who say markets are impossible to time using cycle analysis (discussed in chapter eight) will point out that if you missed the fifty best performance days of the S&P 500 index, you would have damned your portfolio to only a 1.1 percent return for the period between January 4, 1928, and March 10, 1999. (As we all know, when the stock market is bad, it's *really* bad.) If your portfolio could have sidestepped the fifty worst days of S&P 500 performance, it would have performed at a lofty 11.8 percent per year, beating a buy-and-hold strategy return of 6.2 percent by nearly double. So an active strategy makes sense.

As shown in earlier chapters, dividend yields, interest rates, price-earnings ratios, etc, offer ways to identify a cheap (or expensive) market that offers plenty of buying opportunities (or overpriced lemons). Your portfolio should be reviewed annually to ensure that you are structured in a way consistent with a commonsense long-term strategy that emphasizes undervalued investments and avoids overvalued assets. Last, realize there will be periods where any portfolio may significantly underperform certain investment classes due to illogical manias.

# Straight Talk on Growing Old

The overriding premise of this book is to help physicians realize a happy lifetime of financial security for themselves, their spouse, and their dependent children. There are no inventive methods listed to ensure your assets stay intact, by avoiding estate taxes and such, to benefit your children or your children's children after your death. Financial security for you also implies independence so that you avoid being dependent on or a burden to your children. Every physician is aware of the fact that people are living longer. To enjoy life beyond what was formerly considered a normal life expectancy is commonplace today. But with extended life comes new responsibilities, concerns, and issues that must be addressed in any comprehensive retirement plan.

There are more than three million retired US citizens aged eighty-five or older. The US Census Bureau estimates that 18 percent of those people seventy-five to eighty-five years old have trouble walking, and that estimate increases to 35 percent for those over age eighty-five. The reality is that approximately one-third of individuals over seventy-five are living alone but may have one or more living limitations, such as dressing themselves, using the toilet, preparing meals, etc. To physicians who are concerned about never having to count on offspring for support, the reality of the above statistics must be addressed by your retirement plan.

As children, we are dependent on our parents, who nurture and provide for us throughout the years of our education, at which time we become dependent on our skills. By accumulating wealth, we hope to become solely dependent on our investments, but the reality is once again that we will find ourselves dependent on someone else to help us with basic needs. Nursing homes, day nurses, butlers, cooks, maids—a huge industry has arisen to serve the needs of our oldest citizens. For a price, all of your daily living limitations can be taken care of by others. But surprisingly, the cost of assistance is usually much less than the normal costs of retirement. So for the physician who has accumulated a significant retirement nest egg (over $1 million dollars), no special investment account needs to be created for assisted living care.

An additional concern about aging is determining who will make sure you don't inadvertently sell your home, buy into an investment scam, or pay for the newspaper with your private stash of Krugerrands. Who will tell you with honesty and concern that it's logical to have someone assist you with certain responsibilities, even though you feel you are handling them competently?

I encourage you to invite your children, trusted friends, and associates—if they promise always to be honest and objective—to sit down with you once a year to review your finances. I also feel that every advisor you use should be completely trustworthy. Too many physicians handle all the financial concerns, leaving their spouse with very little understanding of the whole picture. Often, these physicians will have advisors they aren't completely sure about, but who provide services that are acceptable because the physician monitors and negotiates each transaction. Such advisors are usually commission-driven stockbrokers, insurance agents, or financial planners positioned to receive commissions for selling products. The danger here, of course, is that, should the physician die and leave the decision-making to the inexperienced spouse, problems might develop.

With the possible exception of your casualty insurance agent, all of your advisors should be fee-only, all the time. Each of your advisors should be willing to give you advice in writing, with additional copies sent to the other advisors in your stable of financial coaches. Hopefully, you will develop a long and rewarding relationship with all your advisors. They should truly feel driven to care about your goals, your family, and any special needs as you grow older.

# The "All Is Well" Talk

Figure 11.1 (Let's Talk Checklist) will help you begin a discussion about personal and financial issues with your loved ones and advisors. Consult with your most trusted financial advisor before diving headlong into a family discussion. Some retirees have given instructions to several advisors/ friends to help monitor their mental health and well-being. They have asked these friends to tell them straight out, "It's time to go in and see if you have Alzheimer's," or to openly discuss any other sensitive subject. Other instructions may include asking to place them as interested parties on investment accounts, checking accounts, credit cards, and other financial accounts.

Furthermore, your spouse should be very familiar with all aspects of your finances and should be included in all meetings with your financial advisors. But ultimately, your financial security is up to you. Only you—with help from trusted advisors—can ensure that "all is well" throughout the duration of your financial life.

**Figure 11.1**

# Let's Talk Checklist

Discuss these issues with your family member(s), fee-only financial planner, CPA, lawyer, and other trusted advisors.

***Wills and trusts:*** Where are they? What do they say?

***Assets:*** What are they? Is there a list of who owns what?

***Goals:***
- Should you die, what (if any) preparations are made for your spouse and/or survivor(s)? Should you become sick?

- Are there daily living limitations that should be addressed (eating, toilet, showering, dressing, etc)?

- Are there special needs for any children due to mental or physical illness, limitations, or the inability to just "grow up and be responsible"?

- Have you made Alzheimer's preparations? Should someone monitor significant purchases; for example, should either spouse sign any checks over $10,000?

- Should kids or a trusted advisor get copies of all portfolio/investment information for monitoring purposes?

- Whom do you or don't you trust?

- Should you develop an incurable disease or become incoherent at the end of your life, who should make end-of-life decisions?

# chapter twelve

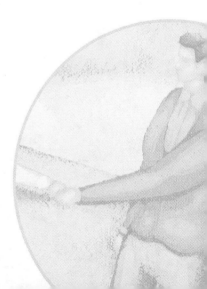

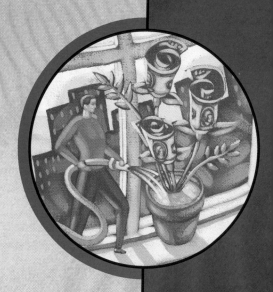

# The Money Is Easy

## Never Too Late

"It is too late!" Ah, nothing is too late—
Cato learned Greek at eighty; Sophocles
wrote his grand "Oedipus," and Simonides
Bore off the prize of verse from his compeers
When each had numbered more than fourscore years;
And Theophrastus, at fourscore and ten,
Had begun his "Characters of Men."
Chaucer, at Woodstock, with his nightingales,
At sixty wrote the "Canterbury Tales."
Goethe, at Weimar, toiling to the last,
Completed "Faust" when eighty years were past.

What then? Shall we sit idly down and say,
"The night has come; it is no longer day?"
For age is opportunity no less
Than youth itself, though in another dress.
And as the evening twilight fades away,
The sky is filled with stars, invisible by day.
It is never too late to start doing what is right.
Never.

—Henry Wadsworth Longfellow (1807–1882)

For many physicians, having plenty of income and financial security is the easy part of retirement, yet there are many other issues and concerns. Depression, anxiety, obsessive behavior, and other ills can befall the retiree who neglects the psychological preparation of ending a career, especially when that career has been as fulfilling as treating pain and sickness. The transition from being a competent, respected, and sought-after professional to a "retired old geezer" can be traumatic, to say the least. One of my clients put it this way: "On Friday I saw forty patients, and on Monday I was following my wife around the house. Only then did I realize that she already had a life. . . . I was a depressed man until I got *it* together."

Every physician's "it" is different. In reality, some physicians should never retire because of the difficulty (impossibility?) of finding some pursuit that replaces the magnitude of their medical life. Regardless of the reasons, there is nothing wrong with working your whole life. Medicine, for many, is not something you do; it is something you are. A sixty-seven-year-old physician client called not long ago and announced that his father had just died. I asked where and how, and he said, "In the operating room; he was in surgery and had a heart attack." He just loved the image of his father putting a scalpel down, sitting down in a chair, and passing away.

# Unhappy at Work

It is also unreasonable to think retirement is going to be easy because you hate your job. But the notion that anything would be better than paperwork, coworkers, getting up at 6:00, on-call duty, those damn new regulations, unappreciative patients, and so on, is dangerously shortsighted. Running away from your job and stumbling into retirement can present many unforeseen problems. Retirement should be something you run toward.

So let's talk about how we can "get it together" in retirement. Many of you may want to skip this information—the psychological cornpone—but I ask kindly that you please bear with me or at least have your spouse read it over.

# The Relaxed Enjoyment of Life

What's a good retirement goal? To pursue a balanced, love-filled, fulfilling, exciting (you fill in the blanks), _____, _____, _____, new life, second life. Or to find that perfect balance among mental, physical, emotional, spiritual, and relationship needs. In other words, to be happy.

Serving others brings with it an accompanying sense of feeling valued, needed, and respected for the years of study and successful practice of combating illness. At the best of times, you might have been happily consumed by your career. Months or years flew by with a great sense of accomplishment.

I believe physicians must pursue retirement as diligently as they pursued their careers. Somehow, somewhere, there must exist a similar feeling of worth to replace the gratification of practicing medicine. It will be different, of course; yet the appetite for the high you knew in medicine must be appeased. Your retirement life might feel like moving to a different country. Can we have a goal of happiness without being able to define happiness?

Like the proverbial questions—"why are we here?" "What gives meaning to life?" "What is a worthy goal?" "What makes life worth living?"—the purpose of retirement is a question that can only be answered individually.

# An Exercise

In retirement you will no longer be a practicing physician, so what are you? How many casual conversations have you found yourself in where the subject of work has come up? Just about all of them, probably. Before you retire, you may find it helpful to practice (while on vacation or on weekends) answering the question "What do you do?" Some potential responses besides "I'm a doctor" may be "Oh, I'm in medicine" or "I'm in business." You might try avoiding the subject altogether by saying "I am husband to my wife and father to my children." Other mildly evasive answers are "I'm learning to be on a vacation" or "When I'm on holiday, I don't like to discuss my work." What do you do? I'm confident you can come up with better answers than "I used to be a physician." Try to feel like you're retired and not a practicing physician any more. Can you do it?

# Diversions and Volunteerism

Throughout this book, we have suggested many ideas for things to do, both now and in retirement. Remember, in your career the goal should be to work when you want, how you want, where you what, and if you want. Try setting a goal of leading a balanced life today. Work on finding enjoyable and fulfilling activities today that you can carry with you into retirement.

*No one should sit down and feel hopeless about problems—there's too much work to be done.*

The volunteer spirit has always run rampant through the medical community. Even now, in these more rigid, turbulent times in health care, physicians continue to donate their special skills to the needy in record numbers. Perhaps no other professional is as valued and indispensable to charitable organizations around the world.

A recent extensive study conducted by Lou Harris Associates found that more than a quarter of the fifty-three million Americans over the age of fifty-five rolled up their sleeves and volunteered in the past year. From

## Resources for Travelers

**National Passport Information Center**
900 225-5674

**Centers for Disease Control**
Information on immunizations necessary
for travel.
www.cdc.gov/

**Up-to-Date International Travel Warnings**
http://travel.state.gov

**Travel & Leisure Magazine**
800 888-8728
www.tlexplorer.com

**Look up average temperature and rainfall
for cities around the world at:**
www.worldclimate.com

**Amtrak Vacation Planner**
Hundreds of US train destinations, including
hotels, tours, rental cars.
888 464-8433

**Geographic Expeditions**
Adventure travel agency with regularly scheduled tours, treks, and safaris to Inner-Asia,
Inner-Africa, Inner-America, Inner-Europe.
800 777-8183
info@geoex.com

**The Online Magazine of European Travel**
www.eurodata.com

**British Footpaths**
914 Mason
Bellingham, WA 98225 USA
360 671-1217
Fax: 360 380-1296
E-mail: bfootpath@aol.com
www.explore-britain.com/footpaths/

**The British Tourist Authority**
www.visitbritain.com

**Castles on the Web**
A Web site entirely devoted to castles in
England, Scotland, or Wales. For example,
typing "Scotland" into your search engine
turns up links to no fewer than twenty-three
Web sites with Scottish castle information.
www.castlesontheweb.com

**LondonNet—The Net Magazine Guide to
London**
What to see and where to stay in London:
news, city guide, accommodations,
entertainment, chat, advice.
http://www.londonnet.co.uk/

**Hostelling International**
Hostelling International (formerly
International Youth Hostels) operates the
world's largest chain of overnight facilities,
with over five thousand hostels in seventy
countries. This page offers the official HI
guidebooks for sale, along with links to
partner organizations around the world.
www.iyhf.org/

**Large directory of hostels**
www.hostels.com

**London Theatre Guide Online**
Very detailed and comprehensive guide to
the London theatre scene, including current
and upcoming productions, reviews, ticket
information (with some special offers), and a
map of London's West End showing the
location of popular theatres.
www.londontheatre.co.uk/

**Theatre Tickets**
This ticket broker for New York, San
Francisco, and London stages also offers
good deals on hotel/theatre packages.
www.theatredirect.com

**Rail Europe**
800 438-7245
www.raileurope.com

## Resources for Travelers *continued*

**Irish Tourist Board**
www.ireland.travel.ie/

**New Zealand Tourism Board**
800 388-5494
www.nztb.govt.nz

**Tourism Offices Worldwide Directory**
www.mbnet.mb.ca/lucas/travel/

**The Universal Currency Converter**
www.xe.net/currency/

**For detailed information on the National Parks of the United States, write to:**
Superintendent of Documents
The Government Printing Office
Washington, DC 20402

***Washington, DC–based Foreign Embassies for Tourist Information:***

| | |
|---|---|
| Australia | 800 242-2878 |
| Bahamas | 202 319-2660 |
| Canada | 202 682-1740 |
| Costa Rica | 202 328-6628 |
| Ecuador (Galapagos Islands) | 202 234-7166 |
| Egypt | 202 895-5400 |
| France | 202 944-6200 |
| Greece | 202 939-5818 |
| India | 202 939-9839 |
| Ireland | 202 462-3939 |
| Italy | 202 328-5500 |
| Jamaica | 202 452-0660 |
| Japan | 202 939-6800 |
| Mexico | 202 736-1000 |
| New Zealand | 202 328-4800 |
| Norway | 202 333-6000 |
| Russia | 202 939-8907 |
| South Africa | 202 966-1650 |
| Spain | 202 728-2330 |
| United Kingdom | 202 588-7800 |

pounding nails to fighting crime, counseling troubled youths in Appalachia to treating the millions of AIDS victims in central Africa as well as in the United States, older Americans are leaving their homes every day to inject a dose of humanity into our world. And what are they getting in return? Simply the intense satisfaction of helping others, of making another person happy. They are serving to remind the impersonal, fax-happy, e-mail-exchanging, techno-faddists in this country how interdependent we all are. Yes, we need each other.

That same Harris Associates survey also indicated that many more older Americans would volunteer if only someone asked them to do so.

A wonderful book titled *Golden Opportunities: A Volunteer Guide for Americans over Fifty* by Andrew Carroll is the veritable end-all resource for wannabe volunteers.* Carroll lists hundreds of organizations—the vast

---

* Andrew Carroll, *Golden Opportunities: A Volunteer Guide for Americans over Fifty* (Princeton, NJ: Peterson's, 1994).

majority for older volunteers—that benefit disadvantaged, oppressed, and just plain needy folk here and around the world. And while different communities have certain, specific needs, special breeds of volunteers are always in demand:

- Volunteers who can work during regular business hours at schools, hospitals, museums, blood centers, etc.
- Volunteers to visit with the residents in nursing homes, chatting, playing cards, writing letters, or just holding a hand.
- Volunteers who can make a long-term commitment (a few hours each week for a year or so) to teach someone how to read, for example.
- Volunteers (especially African American and Latino volunteers) who can mentor children from broken homes.
- Volunteers who can help crisis organizations, like shelters for women or suicide hotlines.
- Volunteers willing to do basic office work—stuffing envelopes, editing newsletters, answering the phone, and so on.

The following list includes organizations specifically looking for physicians and health care professionals to work and volunteer abroad.

**ReliefWeb**
http://wwwnotes.reliefweb.int/
This is a project of the United Nations Office for the Coordination of the Humanitarian Affairs. The Web site contains an extensive list of organizations in need of volunteer assistance.

**American Refugee Committee**
2344 Nicollet Avenue, Suite 350
Minneapolis, MN 55404
612 872-7060

**Christian Medical & Dental Society**
PO Box 7500
Bristol, TN 37620
423 844-1000

**Doctors of the World**
375 West Broadway, 4th Floor
New York, NY 10012
888 817-4357

**Doctors Without Borders USA, Inc**
6 East 39th Street, 8th Floor
New York, NY 10016
888 392-0392

**Doctors Without Borders West**
2040 Avenue of the Stars, 4th Floor
Los Angeles, CA 90067
310 277-2793

**Esperanca**
1911 West Earll Drive,
Phoenix, AZ 85015
602 252-7772

**Health Volunteers Overseas, Inc**
c/o Washington Station, PO Box 65157
Washington, DC 20035-5157
202 296-0928

**International Medical Corps**
11500 West Olympic Boulevard, Suite 506
Los Angeles, CA 90064
800 481-4462

**Interplast**
300-B Pioneer Way
Mountain View, CA 94041-1506
650 962-0123

**Operation Smile**
6435 Tidewater Drive
Norfolk, VA 23509
757 321-7645

**Physicians for Human Rights**
100 Boylston Street, Suite 702
Boston, MA 02116
617 695-0041
www.phrusa.org

**Physicians for Peace Foundation**
229 West Bute Street, Suite 820
Norfolk, VA 23510
757 625-7569

**Project Concern International**
OPTIONS Service
3550 Afton Road
San Diego, CA 92123
619 279-9690

**Project HOPE**
Recruitment Section
Carter Hall
Millwood, VA 22646
800 544-4673 or 703 837-2100

# Suggested Reading

Ferrin, Kelly. *What's Age Got to Do With It?* San Diego, Calif: ALTI Publishing, 1999; ISBN 1-883051-21-5.

Greenwald, Bob. *50 Fabulous Planned Retirement Communities for Active Adults.* Franklin Lakes, NJ: Career Press, 1998; ISBN 1-56414-347-3.

Howells, John. *Where to Retire: America's Best and Most Affordable Places.* Old Saybrook, Conn: The Globe Pequot Press, 1998; ISBN 0-7627-0256-7.

Stern, Ken. *50 Fabulous Places to Retire In America.* Franklin Lakes, NJ: Career Press, 1997; ISBN 1-56414-261-2.

# chapter thirteen

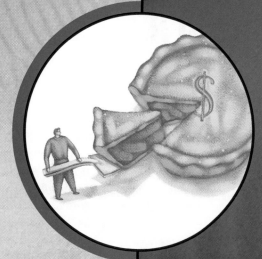

# Estate Planning

**M**illions of dollars are wasted unnecessarily on estate taxes due to poor or inadequate estate planning. (Of course, some people may not see taxes paid after they're dead as a waste.)

Over the years, I have found a majority of physician estate plans to be over-simplified, uncreative, and plain wasteful. Granted, not too many people can get excited about the tedious and complicated project of planning for their own death: *"Your IRA beneficiary designation affects your trust's ability to benefit your will provisions and your Q-TIP trust's provisions to help ensure your kids get something, and their kids get more. But if you forgot to fund your trust—well, that's another matter. Go play tennis or golf and worry about all this later. Your kids and grandkids will be fine after you die."*

Estate planning requires a very competent CPA-attorney combination with the patience to listen to you describe your goals and then explain to you hundreds of options. The one issue you should keep in mind as you start wading into the estate planning waters is that if you do things right—before you die—your spouse will receive all of your assets tax-free when you do die, whether there is $100,000 or $100 million or more. Simply by making a beneficiary designation, a will, and a trust, you can ensure your spouse (not attorneys or the government) will get it all. Beyond that, taking care of your kids and grandkids is more complicated and requires solid estate planning advice. Here are some basics that will help you have a reasonable conversation with your attorney or CPA estate planner.

> **The average fee-only financial advisor serving physicians found that . . .**
> Their average retired client has $1 million to $3.8 million in retirement assets.

# Wills, Trusts, and Other Estate Planning Tools

A will contains directions for the administration and disposition of your estate following your death. It enables a person to set forth his or her wishes as to how the estate will be probated, and to whom and when that estate will be distributed. Probate is the process that ensures that the wishes expressed in the will are carried out. The act of having a will prepared for you (and signing it) means you are not restricted in terms of ownership, administration, or disposition of any of the assets that you own. Your will, if prepared according to applicable state law, does not become effective until your death.

A trust is a separate legal entity that you create by means of a trust document, either separately or as a part of your will. The trust may be in the form of a "testamentary" trust (part of your will) and comes into existence following your death and after the probate of your estate. Trusts may also take the form of a living trust (separate from your will), sometimes referred to as a revocable living (or loving) trust and one that is funded during your lifetime.

The revocable living trust will not be probated at the time of your death because the trust is a separate legal entity, and its existence continues after your death. A living trust allows you control over the trust assets and administration; you can name yourself as trustee and administer the trust assets during your lifetime, with a successor trustee named in the document to take over the administration of the trust assets immediately upon your death.

The trust can also be used to reduce estate taxes (following your death) by dividing your estate into separate shares for surviving spouse and children (family and marital trusts). The trust, whether a living trust or a testamentary trust, may be designed simply for the purpose of receiving insurance proceeds following your death. It will contain directions for administration and distribution of those proceeds.

An irrevocable trust may be appropriate if one of your objectives is to remove assets from your estate for the benefit of other beneficiaries without an immediate outright distribution to those beneficiaries. You may also accomplish estate reduction by means of gifts; if these gifts are less than $10,000 per donee, they will not incur a gift tax. If the gifts are to charitable, religious, educational, or similar organizations, they may also qualify for the income tax charitable deduction (not usually subject to an amount limitation).

Another important estate planning tool is the durable power of attorney. This is a document wherein you designate someone as your "attorney-in-fact" and give them the power to handle your business affairs. They may also make personal decisions for you in the event that you become incompetent. A durable power of attorney is valid only during your lifetime, and any authority granted in that document terminates upon your death. It can allow you to avoid the involvement of a probate court, establishing a guardianship or conservatorship to supervise the administration of your estate, including helping you make personal decisions, during your period of incompetency. In addition to preparing for death legally, prepare your family emotionally. I also suggest to my clients that they write a letter to the "key players," outlining their wishes and how they are to be carried out.

# Trusts, Trustees, and Who Should Handle Assets

After naming guardians, the second hardest decision for most people in their estate plan is deciding who should be the trustee to administer the trust (make sure that your wishes are carried out). We have all heard distressing stories about local trust companies being purchased by regional trust companies, only to be swallowed up by yet another larger regional bank. Suddenly, the trust officer is a three-hour flight away, and assets are being handled by a faceless manager. I have heard of people having as many as eight different trust officers in a period of two years.

To avoid these situations, it is always best to have a trusted friend (or a number of dependable friends) as cotrustee(s) to work with the corporate trustee. Only one-third of the trusts administered in the United States are trusteed by corporate trustees, so don't feel compelled to use their services. Once you find a trustee that knows your children, knows the beneficiary of your trust, and is one that you trust implicitly, make sure that you leave that person enough instructions (through the trust document, a specific letter to them, and thorough discussions) so that they feel very comfortable administering your trust. You might suggest a money manager you think would be appropriate to manage the assets in your trust or name a CPA or accounting firm to administer the trust.

Be cautious and very thorough. If the trust states that the trustees have the ability to send the child to college, does that mean that the child can go to Harvard? Does that mean the child can pursue a doctorate? These things need to be stated in the trust or in a letter to the trustee to facilitate interpretation of the finer points. Keep in mind that while your beneficiaries know who you set the trust up for, they usually have no say in how the trust is managed. While you may be enamored of the local trust agent because of the wonderful services at the bank, your heirs may later find out that those who set up the trust at the corporate level have been replaced. Or they could find that the personal investment management services of your trust company have funneled all the funds into one of the bank's mediocre performance mutual funds, and they have charged you not only a trust administration fee but also a fee on the mutual fund. Always allow your beneficiaries the right to change trust companies or change trustees, with restrictions that do not violate trust laws. Your financial counselors can help you with this point.

Another easy method of avoiding conflict between your current trusted beneficiaries and your subsequent heirs is to name specific amounts of money rather than the more common arrangement where trustees will send out all the income generated in the trust. The trustee could buy 2 percent dividend-yielding stocks or 8 percent interest-bearing bonds. The 2 percent common stocks would probably be much better for whomever ultimately receives the corpus of your trust, but if your goal is current income, the bonds are a better choice. Thus, it is a good idea to always name fixed dollar or percentage amounts in your trust. For example, a savvy trust would state that income beneficiaries receive 6 percent of the trust corpus per year as income. Whatever is left goes to the ultimate beneficiaries.

Naturally, it is appropriate to put in inflation adjustments whenever you put specific numbers in the document. If you use a corporate trustee, it is also appropriate to state that any legal fees paid to defend the trustees are not paid out of your trust but instead are paid by the trust company. If you use a corporate trustee or are a beneficiary of a corporate trust, make sure that you enlighten your financial advisors when matters concerning the trust come up. In this way, they can be looking over your trustee's shoulder to make sure things are going appropriately.

Figure 13.1 (Estate Planning List) summarizes some of the things to do to make your family aware of your plans.

For more information on estate planning, I recommend these two books:

Condon, Gerald M, and Jeffrey L Condon. *Beyond the Grave: The Right and the Wrong Way of Leaving Money to Your Children (and Others)*. New York: HarperBusiness, 1995.

Kubicek, Theodore L. *Your Worldly Possessions: A Complete Guide to Preserving, Passing On, and Inheriting Property*. Burr Ridge, Ill: McGraw-Hill), 1992.

# Event-Driven Dispositions

If you knew that in five years you were going to receive two million dollars, would it change your behavior now? Would your behavior change if you knew (at age eighteen) that you would receive half a million dollars at age twenty-five, the same amount at thirty, and a million dollars at thirty-five? In all probability, you would not be in the position you are in today.

Knowing that, most people still set up age-driven dispositions in their trusts. A saner way of distributing assets to heirs is under what I call "event-driven dispositions." Perhaps you set up a trust to pay for all your children's college expenses and provide them with a one thousand dollar monthly stipend for food, books, travel, and extra expenses. The big carrot is that your children will receive the lump sum when they graduate.

**Figure 13.1**

# Estate Planning List

1. Your spouse (or father, mother, siblings, children, friends, etc) should know whom to call if you die, and where to find a list of your assets and important papers.

2. Your spouse should have a letter of instructions and suggestions of whom you feel should be trusted as an advisor for:

   a. Accounting

   b. Legal work

   c. Investment advice

   d. Insurance

   e. General financial planning help

3. Your spouse should know your specific wishes concerning funeral details, including: cremation, burial, organ gifting, and cemetery choice.

4. Your children should know whom you have named as guardians and why you chose those particular people.

5. You should have a "letter of values" written to your chosen guardians, stating why you picked them to care for your children. In addition, the letter should state your child-rearing values and beliefs on schooling, sports, colleges, summer camps, driving, travel, visiting relatives, etc. (A similar letter should go to your trustees.)

Instead, you could structure the disposition so that your children get one-fifth of the trust in a lump sum of money when they receive their undergraduate degree, another fifth when they get their graduate degree, and maybe the balance in a lump sum. Other "incentive events" are postdoctorate degrees, birth of a child, marriage, purchase of a first home, venture capital for starting a business, or completion of a stint in the Peace Corps. Some documents simply allow the trustee to match the earned income of the beneficiary. Most attorneys are quite unimaginative when it comes to estate planning and will generally try to place you in a box with no room for creativity in your plan.

Other interesting ideas I have seen in trusts include these: (1) The children are allowed to direct a certain amount of money to a charity each month; (2) funds are provided for a regular family gathering; (3) lump sums are provided to travel the world or make a special trip to a specific destination.

The most important thing to remember about your trust and estate plan is that it should be personal. It should reflect *your* values, not the values of your lawyer, accountant, or any other advisor. This could be the most important document you will ever draft, so think about it and think creatively. Don't worry about the tax issues; worry about what you want for your family should something happen to you. Be aware that preparing your estate documents will take time and emotional energy, but the payoff to your family's future will be immeasurable.

# glossary

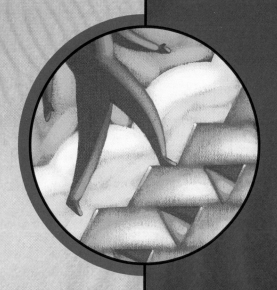

**AARP:** American Association of Retired Persons.

**Administrator:** Individual or entity who is selected to be responsible for reporting to and complying with all Internal Revenue Service and Department of Labor requirements in the administration of retirement plans.

**Agent:** One who acts for another, called a principal. One who represents another from whom he has derived authority.

**Aggressive Growth Fund:** A stock-oriented mutual fund with an investment objective of substantial capital gains and little income over the long term.

**Annual Mutual Fund Expense Ratio:** Yearly mutual fund fee assessed to cover the fund's expenses, including management fees, transaction fees, and marketing expenses. Annual expense ratios usually vary from .20 percent to about 3 percent of a fund's net asset value. The expense ratio is deducted from each shareholder's holdings.

**Annual Renewable Term (ART):** A form of pure protection life insurance that guarantees the right to renew coverage each year without evidence of insurability (physical examination), usually to age sixty-five.

**Annual Report:** The formal financial and important information statement issued yearly by a corporation, trust, or other entity. The annual report shows assets, liabilities, earnings, standing of the company at the close of the business year, performance of the company profitwise during the year, and other information of interest to share owners.

**Annuity:** A retirement vehicle that provides for the payment of a specific sum of money at uniform intervals of time (usually monthly). It provides the annuitant with a guaranteed income either immediately or at retirement. Annuities usually pay until death (or for a specific period of time) and provide protection against the possibility of outliving your financial resources.

**Arbitrage:** Dealing in differences. *Example:* buying on one exchange while simultaneously selling short on another market at a higher price.

**ASCLU:** American Society of Chartered Life Underwriters (insurance agents).

**Asset:** On a balance sheet, that which is owned or receivable.

**Back-End Load:** A commission/fee charged investors by some commission broker–sold mutual funds when the investors sell their shares in the fund. The fees, which range from about 1 percent to 6 percent, typically reduce by about 1 percent each year the investor holds the fund. For instance, a fund with a maximum 5 percent back-end load will charge the full 5 percent the first year. But the fee normally drops to 4 percent the second year, 3 percent the third, 2 percent the fourth, 1 percent the fifth, and zero after the fifth year. The two types of back-end loads are *deferred sales charges* and *redemption fees*. Funds with deferred sales fees base charges on the net asset value of the shares when they were purchased, whereas redemption fees are based on the price of the shares at the time they are sold. Thus, if a fund has a strong gain, much more is paid in redemption fees than in deferred sales charges. Back-end loads are a bad deal; avoid funds with back-end loads. (See also: **Load, No-Load, Front-End Load, Redemption Fee**, and **Deferred Sales Charge**)

**Balanced Fund:** A mutual fund that is required to keep within a specified percentage range of its total assets invested in senior securities, like bonds.

**Bargain Investment:** An investment that appears to be at a low price and, thus, a bargain when compared to its earnings and earning power potential, price-to-assets, franchise value, and relative attractiveness within its market. Usually bargain hunter investors scour the world for investments that are neglected or out of favor, in other words, bargains because the perception of them differs from the reality.

**Bear:** Someone who believes the market will decline.

**Bear Market:** A declining market.

**Beneficiary:** A person designated by a participant in a retirement plan or one who, by the terms of the plan, is or becomes eligible for benefits under the plan. For life insurance, the person, trust, corporation, etc, named to receive proceeds at death.

**Bid and Asked:** Often referred to as a quotation or quote. The bid is the highest price anyone has declared that he wants to pay for a security at a given time; the asked is the lowest price anyone will take at the same time. The difference is the spread.

**Big Board:** Term for the New York Stock Exchange, Inc.

**Blind Pool Program:** A *tax-sheltered program* which, at the time sale of *subscriptions* begins, does not have much proceeds of the offering allocated to specific purposes, projects, or properties. These are usually higher risk due to their dependence on management.

**Block:** A large holding or transaction of stock, usually 10,000 shares or more.

**Blue Chip:** A company known nationally for its products or services and for its ability to make money and pay dividends. Large companies that make up the Dow Jones Average or large S&P 500 companies are often considered blue chips.

**Bond:** Basically, debt issued by a government or corporations, usually issued in multiples of $1,000. A bond usually promises to pay the bondholders a specified amount of interest for a specified length of time, and to repay the loan on the expiration date. In every case, a bond represents debt; its holder is a creditor of the corporation and not a part owner, as is the shareholder.

**Bond Fund:** A mutual fund invested primarily in bonds.

**Book Value:** An accounting term for the valuation of a stock determined from a company's records by adding all assets and then deducting all debts and other liabilities, plus the liquidation price of any preferred issues. The sum arrived at is divided by the number of common shares outstanding, and the result is book value per common share.

**Bottom Up:** An investment method in which an investor selects stocks based on the merits of each individual investment, without regard to the overall economy. This is the opposite of a top-down approach, in which an investor looks at broad economic patterns to determine which investment sectors to buy or avoid. (See also: **Top Down**)

**Broker:** An agent who handles the public's orders to buy and sell securities, commodities, or other property. A commission, markup, or other fee is charged for this service.

**Bull:** One who believes the stock market will rise.

**Bull Market:** An advancing stock market.

**Business Cycle:** The normal, long-term, economic boom-recession cycle that has been characteristic of the fluctuations in employment, growth, and other business conditions not only nationally, but worldwide.

**Call:** An option to buy a specified number of shares of a certain security at a certain price within a specified period of time.

**Callable:** A bond or preferred stock issue, all or part of which may be redeemed by the issuing corporation or government under specific conditions before maturity.

**Cannibalizing Assets:** Funds that pay part of their distributions out of principal cannibalize their assets. This depletes the fund's asset base. Funds cannibalize assets to maintain a dividend and keep shareholders happy. However, like feeding a cow its own milk, this practice cannot go on forever.

**Capital Gain** or **Capital Loss:** Profit or loss from the sale of a capital investment asset.

**CEBS:** Certified Employee Benefits Specialist (employee benefits).

**CFP:** Certified Financial Planner (financial planning).

**Charitable Remainder Trust:** A trust where income usually goes to its grantor(s) and at death donates the principal to a charity.

**ChFC:** Chartered Financial Consultant (insurance).

**CIC:** Certified Insurance Counselor.

**Classes of Mutual Fund Shares:** Some mutual fund companies issue fund shares with several pricing classifications. The shares, which normally are referred to as "A" class, "B" class, "C" class, "D" class, and so on, usually have the same portfolio mix but different investor charges. For instance, A shares may have a front-end sales load and a lower annual expense ratio, whereas B shares may have a back-end load and a slightly higher annual expense ratio, C shares may have no sales load but a very high annual expense ratio, and D shares may be geared to institutional and affluent investors with very low fees and may require a minimum investment of $100,000 or more.

**CLU:** Chartered Life Underwriter (insurance).

**COLA:** Cost-of-Living Adjustment.

**College for Financial Planning:** An organization that offers professional training leading to the granting of the CFP designation (Certified Financial Planner). The courses include financial planning, risk management, investments, tax planning, retirement, and estate planning, among others.

**Commission:** The salesperson's or broker's fee for purchasing or selling securities, property, or insurance for a client.

**Commodities:** Real/hard assets and other staple products that are usually traded in bulk form. Examples include platinum, corn, copper, meats, and lumber.

**Common Stocks:** Certificates representing an undivided ownership interest in the assets of a corporation with no predetermined set rate of return. Ownership of common stock provides for corporate voting rights and an interest/share of the future profit (or loss) of the company.

**Compensation:** Compensation paid to a retirement plan's participant is the basic factor that employers use to determine the amount of contributions that will be allocated to a participant's account under a defined contribution plan (eg, a profit-sharing plan) or the amount of benefits that a participant will receive upon retirement. The term is usually broadly defined in the plan to include, but is not limited to, base salary, commissions, bonuses, overtime, and vacation pay. The IRS requires that the definition used in the retirement plan not be discriminatory (ie, favoring highly compensated employees over lower-paid employees). Further, a ceiling may apply to the amount of compensation that may be taken into account under certain types of plans. For IRA purposes, taxable alimony is treated as compensation.

**Compound Interest:** Interest computed on principal plus interest accrued during a previous period or periods. Interest may be computed daily, monthly, quarterly, or semiannually for compounding purposes.

**Continuing Care (Life Care) Community:** A retirement facility in which residents can lead active lives for as long as they're able, get help when they need it, and receive full-time nursing care if that becomes necessary. A large up-front fee, or endowment, plus monthly fees are usually required.

**Convertible Term Insurance:** An option offered with some term insurance policies that allows the insured to convert the term policy to a universal or whole life policy at some future date.

**Cooperative Apartment:** A housing unit within a building containing other units. A co-op owner owns a share of a certain percentage of the entire property, which gives the owner the right to live in one of the units.

**Corporation:** A group or body of persons established and treated by law as an individual or unit with rights and liabilities or both, distinct and apart from the persons composing it.

**Cost-of-Living Adjustments (COLA):** Adjustments that are made annually by the IRS to the limitations on maximum benefits and maximum contributions to retirement plans that could be made to a qualified pension or profit-sharing plan for a particular taxable year. Also has to do with Social Security and other pension adjustments due to inflation's effect on the cost of living.

**CPA:** Certified Public Accountant (accountant).

**CPC:** Certified Pension Consultant (pension plans).

**Custodian:** Any person or organization holding the assets of another. Also used to refer to an adult who agrees to take responsibility for a minor or to a bank that serves as a depository for the assets of an IRA or mutual fund.

**DB Plans:** Defined benefit retirement plans.

**Death Benefits:** Payments to a beneficiary of a deceased participant that may be provided under an insurance policy, qualified retirement plan, etc.

**Debenture:** A promissory note backed by the general credit of a company and usually not secured by a mortgage or lien on any specific property.

**Debit Card:** A charge card where no credit is issued that is used like a "plastic check." Issued by some bank holding companies, money market funds, and MasterCard and Visa. Amounts of purchases made with the debit card are deducted the same day from a cardholder's money market, checking, or savings account.

**Decreasing Term:** A type of pure protection life insurance (term) in which the premiums remain the same and face value of coverage decreases over the life of the policy.

**Deduction:** Any reduction of taxable income that ultimately reduces the amount of tax due.

**Deferral:** A form of tax shelter resulting from an investment that is timed so deductions take place during the investor's high-income years; hopefully, capital gains or other income take place after retirement or in some other period of reduced income tax liability.

**Deferred Annuity:** An annuity issued by an insurance company in which income payments begin in the future (specified age or stated number of years).

**Deferred Sales Charge:** An unnecessary commission/sales fee, often called a "back-end load," charged shareholders by some mutual funds when the shareholders sell their fund shares (a way of "hiding" the commission). (See **Back-End Load**)

**Defined Benefit Plan:** A type of qualified retirement plan that determines a participant's benefit based on a preset benefit formula that assumes the participant will continue to work until retirement age.

**Depreciation:** Normally, charges against earnings to write off the cost, less salvage value, of an asset over its estimated useful life. A bookkeeping entry, it does not represent any cash outlay.

**Director:** A person elected by stockholders or shareholders to establish company policies. The directors elect the president, vice president, and all other operating officers. Directors decide, among other matters, if and when dividends will be paid.

**Discount:** (1) The amount by which a preferred stock or bond may sell below its par value. (2) Refers to a closed-end fund trading at a market price below its net asset value.

**Discount Broker:** A securities or real estate broker who provides lower rates compared to those for full services.

**Discretionary Account:** An investment account in which the customer gives an investment advisor, lawyer, broker, or someone else discretion, either complete or within specific limits, as to the purchase and sale of real estate, securities, commodities, or other assets, including selection, timing, amount, and price to be paid or received.

**Discretionary Formula Plan:** A profit-sharing retirement plan which provides that the amount of each year's contribution will be determined by the board of directors (or responsible official[s]) of the sponsoring employer, in its discretion. (Contributions must be "recurring and substantial" to keep the plan in a qualified status.)

**Discrimination:** Where a retirement or other employee benefit plan, through its provisions or through its operations, favors officers, shareholders, or highly compensated employees to the detriment of other employees.

**Disqualification:** Loss of qualified (tax-favored) status by a retirement plan, generally resulting from operation of the plan in a manner that is contrary to the provisions of the plan or that discriminates against rank-and-file employees. (See also: **Discrimination**)

**Diversification:** Allocating a portfolio's resources among different investments to reduce the risk of losses that would affect the portfolio's overall returns over time.

**Dividend:** The payment designated by the board of directors to be distributed pro rata among the shares outstanding. On preferred shares, it is generally a fixed amount. On common shares, the dividend varies and may be omitted if business is poor or the directors determine to withhold earnings to invest in plant and equipment. Sometimes a company will pay a dividend out of past earnings even if it is not currently operating at a profit. Mutual funds holding dividend-paying stocks pass those dividends on to shareholders in lump sum payments either monthly, quarterly, semiannually, or annually, depending on the fund. Investors in most funds may have the option to have dividends automatically reinvested in additional shares.

**Dividend Reinvestment Plan:** A mutual fund share account in which dividends are automatically reinvested in additional shares. With this type of account, capital gains distributions are also automatically reinvested.

**Dividend Yield:** The annual dividend payment divided by the market price per share. If a stock is trading at $10 a share and it pays a $.50 dividend, the dividend yield is 5 percent.

**DOL:** Department of Labor. The nontax (regulatory and administrative) provisions of ERISA are administered by the Department of Labor. The department issues opinion letters and other pronouncements affecting employee benefit plans like retirement plans and requires certain information forms to be filed.

**Dollar-Cost-Averaging:** A system of buying specific securities at specific, regular intervals with a fixed dollar amount. Under this system, the investor buys by the dollars' worth rather than by the number of shares. If each investment is of the same number of dollars, payments buy more when the price is low and fewer when it rises. Temporary downswings in price thus benefit the investor if he or she continues to make periodic purchases in both good times and bad, and the price at which the shares are sold is usually more than their average cost.

**Double Taxation:** The federal government taxes corporate profits first as corporate income; any part of the remaining profits distributed as dividends to stockholders may be taxed again as income to the stockholder.

**Earmarking:** Allowing a participant in a defined contribution plan to direct the investment of her or his account.

**Employee:** An individual who provides services to an employer for compensation and whose duties are under the control of the employer.

**Equity (Stocks):** The ownership interest of common and preferred stockholders in a company. Also refers to excess of value of securities over the debit balance in a margin account. Also the value of a property that remains after all liens and other charges against the property are paid.

**Equity Investment:** A security (usually common stock, convertibles, warrants, or convertible preferred stock) that represents a share of ownership in a business entity (usually a corporation).

**ERISA:** Employee Retirement Income Security Act of 1974. This is the basic law covering qualified plans and incorporates both the pertinent Internal Revenue Code provisions and labor law provisions.

**Estate:** All of a person's owned property.

**Estate Planning:** A system of planning designed to ensure your estate will go to whom you want with confidentiality, limited red tape, and the most favorable tax treatment.

**Estate Tax:** A tax assessed on the transfer of wealth in an estate.

**Event Risk:** An unexpected occurrence, like a leveraged buyout, that reduces the creditworthiness of a company's debt, causing its bond prices to drop sharply.

**Exclusive Benefit Rule:** Retirement plan fiduciaries must discharge their duties solely in the interest of participants and beneficiaries for the exclusive purpose of providing benefits to participants and beneficiaries and paying administration expenses. (See also: **Fiduciary**)

**Executor:** A person named in a will to carry out the provisions of the will.

**Face Value:** Face value is ordinarily the amount the issuing company promises to pay at maturity of a bond. Face value is not an indication of market value. It is sometimes called par value.

**Family of Funds:** A system of mutual funds, managed by the same company, that provides the option of switching investments from one type of fund to another, either for free or for a small fee.

**Family Trust:** A trust that provides income to a spouse and, upon the spouse's death, is automatically disbursed to children.

**Federal Deposit Insurance Corporation (FDIC):** A corporation established by federal authority to provide insurance on demand and time deposits in participating banks up to a maximum of $100,000 for each depositor.

**Fee and Commission Advisor:** An investment or financial advisor that can receive commissions in addition to receiving or charging fees. This advisor usually emphasizes his or her ability to be objective by charging a fee for the advice, but it's usually found that recommendations line the pocket of the fee plus commission adviser.

**Fee-Based Advisor:** Same as a fee and commission advisor; however, the term "sounds better" than "fee and commission" advisor.

**Fee-Only Advisor:** A common term for an investment or financial advisor who believes that commissions "taint" an advisor's objectivity and, thus, cause her or his advice to be less efficient and/or more costly. A fee-only advisor refuses any and all commissions or remuneration from any one other than the investor/client. The National Association of Personal Financial Advisors (NAPFA) champions the fee-only approach as the best deal for the consumer.

**Fiduciary:** A person who exercises any discretionary authority or control over the management or disposition of a retirement plan's assets or gives investment advice to the plan. Any person who renders advice, management, or assistance in regard to a qualified retirement plan is a fiduciary.

**Forfeitures:** The benefits that a participant loses if she or he terminates her or his employment before becoming eligible for full retirement benefits under the retirement plan. For example, a participant who leaves the service of an employer at a time when she or he will receive only 60 percent of her or his benefits forfeits the remaining 40 percent. Under a profit-sharing plan, forfeitures are usually allocated among the remaining participants. Under a defined benefit, money purchase, or target benefit pension plan, the forfeitures are used to reduce employer contributions.

**401k Plan:** A type of profit-sharing plan that allows employees to set aside for retirement part of their gross pay (maximum $9,500) before-tax, into a tax-deferred trust until it is withdrawn.

**Free/Commission-Based Advisor:** Some commissioned salespeople will charge no fee for their advice, saying it's free, but expecting that financial products will be purchased from her or him to compensate the salesperson for their time.

**Front-End Load:** The sales fee a mutual fund charges investors to buy shares of the fund. The commission (usually in the range of 3 percent to 8.5 percent) is deducted directly from the investor's contribution to be paid to the broker and for other marketing costs. For instance, a $1,000 investment in a fund with a 5 percent front-end load would result in $50 in load fees and $950 in actual fund shares.

**Frozen Plan:** A qualified pension or profit-sharing plan that continues to exist even though employer contributions have been discontinued and benefits are no longer accrued by participants. The plan is "frozen" for purposes of distribution of benefits under the terms of the plan.

**FSA:** Fellow of Society of Actuaries (pension plans).

**Fully Managed Fund:** A mutual fund whose investment policy gives its management complete flexibility as to the types of investments made and the proportions of each. Management is restricted only to the extent that federal or state laws require.

**General Partner:** The individual (or individuals) who has unlimited liability in a partnership. Usually distinguished from a limited partner in a real estate, hedge fund, or tax-shelter investment.

**Gift Tax:** A tax levied on the transfer of property as a gift. Paid by the giver or donor.

**Group Living:** An arrangement whereby a group of persons rent or buy a dwelling and share equally in expenses. Sometimes a community sponsors the arrangement and a paid professional supervises the running of the household.

**Government Bonds:** Obligations of a government, regarded as the highest-grade issues in existence, naturally dependent on country of issue.

**Growth Fund:** A mutual fund with an investment objective of capital growth and capital gains. Usually, a common stock fund seeking long-term capital growth and future income rather than current income, with little regard to short-term volatility.

**Growth Investments:** Usually include (growth stock) mutual funds, raw land, collectibles, equities, and stocks, among others.

**Growth Stock:** One of the two types of common stock. Growth stocks seek selling price increases rather than income in the form of dividends for shareholders. (See **Income Stock**)

**Guaranteed Renewable:** An insurance policy renewable at the option of the insured to a stated age, usually sixty or sixty-five.

**Hard Assets:** Investments that are tangible, like precious metals, gems, art, stamps, collectibles, etc.

**Home Sharing:** An arrangement where older homeowners are matched with a "sharer-renter," who shares living expenses and/or provides services.

**Income Fund:** A mutual fund with an investment objective of current income rather than capital growth. Bond funds are considered income funds.

**Income Stock:** One of the two types of common stock. Income stocks seek current income rather than selling price increases or capital growth. (See **Growth Stock**)

**Inflation:** An economic condition of increasing prices.

**Integrated Plan:** A retirement plan that takes into account either benefits or contributions under Social Security. Social Security benefits are used to integrate a defined benefit plan, while Social Security contributions are used with defined contribution plans.

**Intrinsic Value** or **Investment Value:** What an investment is really worth independent of its current market price. Intrinsic value is the end product of the fundamental analysis of a company.

**Investment:** The use of money for the purpose of making more money: to gain income or increase capital or both.

**Investment Advisor:** A broad term used to describe a professional who is selected to manage investments, usually regulated by the Securities & Exchange Commission.

**Investment Club:** A way to join with other novice investors and pool small dollar amounts to buy stocks and learn more about the stock market at the same time.

**Investment Counsel:** One whose principal business consists of acting as investment advisor and rendering investment supervisory services.

**Investment Manager:** Investment portfolio fiduciary who has the power to manage, acquire, or dispose of investments in the portfolio.

**Investor:** An individual whose principal concerns in the purchase of a security usually are income, safety of investment, and capital appreciation.

**IRA:** Individual Retirement Account.

**IRS:** Internal Revenue Service.

**JD:** Doctor of Jurisprudence (attorney).

**Joint and Survivor Annuity:** An annuity paid for the life of the retirement participant with a survivor annuity for her or his spouse. The survivor annuity must be at least 50 percent, but not more than 100 percent, of the annuity received by the participant during her or his lifetime. Also, the joint and survivor annuity must be the actuarial equivalent of a single life annuity that would have been paid to the participant.

**Joint and Two-Thirds Survivor Annuity:** An annuity under which joint annuitants receive payments during a joint lifetime. After the demise of one of the annuitants, the other receives two-thirds of the annuity payments in effect during the joint lifetime.

**Keogh Plan:** A qualified retirement plan, either a defined contribution plan or a defined benefit plan, that is available to self-employed persons and their employees.

**Land Contract:** A form of creative finance used in real estate wherein the seller retains legal title to the property until the buyer makes an agreed-upon number of payments to the seller.

**Lease:** A contract similar to renting between owner and user of the asset, setting forth conditions upon which lessor may use the property, stating terms of the lease.

**Level Term:** A form of pure protection insurance (term) in which the face value and the premiums remain level for a certain period or the life of the policy.

**Leverage:** The effect on the per share earnings of the common stock of a company when large sums must be paid for bond interest or preferred stock dividends or both before the common stock is entitled to share in earnings. Leverage is risky but may be advantageous for the common stock when earnings are good; however, it will work against the common stock holders when earnings decline. Leverage also refers to the amount of debts compared to the income and assets of people or businesses.

**Limited Partner:** In this context, a participant in a *hedge fund* or *venture* that has been organized as a *limited partnership* (See **Limited Partnership**)

**Limited Partnership:** A form of business organization in which some partners exchange their right to participate in management for a limitation on their liability for partnership losses. Commonly, *limited partners* have liability only to the extent of their investment in the venture. To establish limited liability, there must be at least one *general partner* who is fully liable for all claims against the business. A limited partnership is a popular organizational form for *tax-sheltered programs* because of the ease with which tax benefits flow through the partnership to the individual partners.

**Liquidity:** The ability of the market in a particular security to absorb a reasonable amount of buying or selling at reasonable price changes. Liquidity is one of the most important characteristics of a good market.

**Listed Stock:** The stock of a company that is traded on a securities exchange and for which a listing application and a registration statement, giving detailed information about the company and its operations, have been filed with the Securities & Exchange Commission, unless otherwise exempted, and the exchange itself.

**Load:** A commission sales fee charged to mutual fund investors who buy load funds. Loads normally vary from about 3 percent to 8.5 percent of the total purchase amount.

**Long:** Signifies "ownership" of securities. "I am long 100 Merck" means you own 100 shares of Merck.

**Management Fee:** The fee paid to the investment manager of a mutual fund or portfolio. It is usually about one-half of 1 percent to 1.5 percent of average net assets annually. Not to be confused with a mutual fund's sales charge, which is the commission charged on some funds.

**Margin Call:** A demand upon a customer to put up money or securities with the broker. The call is made when a purchase is made or when a customer's equity in a margin account declines below a minimum standard set by the exchange or by the firm.

**Market Capitalization:** The total market value of a publicly traded company; it equals the product of its per share price and the number of shares outstanding. For example, a company selling at $10 per share with 10 million shares outstanding would have a market capitalization or total market value of $100 million.

**Market Multiple:** The price-earnings ratio (or P/E) for the overall market as measured, for example, by the P/E for Standard & Poor's 500 Index or Dow Index. The market multiple provides an important indicator of the overall level of stock values.

**Market Order:** An order to buy or sell a stated amount of a security at the most advantageous price obtainable.

**Market Price:** In the case of a security, market price is usually considered the last reported price at which the stock or bond sold.

**Maturity:** The date on which a loan or a bond becomes due and is to be paid off.

**MBA:** Master of Business Administration (advanced business degree).

**Minimum Funding:** The minimum amount that must be contributed by an employer that has a defined benefit, money purchase, or target benefit pension plan. The minimum is made up of amounts that go to cover "normal costs" (for the benefits earned by employees for the current year) plus other plan liabilities, such as "past service costs"—liabilities for benefits that have been earned for services performed prior to the adoption of the plan. If the employer fails to meet these minimum standards, in the absence of a waiver from the IRS, an excise tax will be imposed on the amount of the deficiency.

**Money Market Fund:** A mutual fund that invests in high-quality, short-term debt instruments such as Treasury bills, commercial paper, and/or certificates of deposit. Money market fund investors earn a steady stream of interest income that varies with short-term interest rates and generally may cash out at any time.

**Money Purchase Pension Plan:** A defined contribution pension plan in which the employer must contribute a certain percentage of each employee's salary each year, regardless of the company's profit.

**Mortgage:** An instrument by which the borrower (mortgagor) gives the lender (mortgagee) a lien on real estate as security for a loan. The borrower, while owning, can use the property, and when the loan is repaid, the lien is removed or satisfied.

**Mortgage Bond:** A bond secured by a mortgage on a property. The value of the property may or may not equal the value of the so-called mortgage bonds issued against it.

**Municipal Bond:** A bond issued by a state or a political subdivision, such as a county, city, town, or village. The term also designates bonds issued by state agencies and authorities. In general, interest paid on municipal bonds is exempt from federal income taxes and from state and local income taxes within the state of issue.

**Mutual Fund:** Usually considered an open-end registered investment company that continuously offers to sell new mutual fund shares to the public in addition to redeeming its shares on demand as required by law. (The term *mutual fund* has no meaning in law.)

**NAPFA:** National Association of Personal Financial Advisors; fee-only financial advisors with very strict member requirements.

**NASD:** National Association of Securities Dealers, Inc, is an association of brokers and dealers in the over-the-counter securities business. The association has the power to expel members who have been declared guilty of unethical practices. NASD is dedicated to, among other objectives, "adopt, administer and enforce rules of fair practice and rules to prevent fraudulent and manipulative acts and practices, and in general to promote just and equitable principles of trade for the protection of investors."

**NASDAQ:** National Association of Securities Dealers Automated Quotations; an automated information network that provides brokers and dealers with price quotations on securities traded over-the-counter.

**Net Asset Value:** A term usually used in connection with investment companies (mutual funds), meaning net asset value per share. It is common practice for a mutual fund to compute its assets daily by totaling the market value of all securities owned. All liabilities are deducted, and the balance is divided by the number of shares outstanding. The resulting figure is the net asset value per share.

**Net Change:** The change in the price of a security from the closing price on one day to the closing price on the following day on which the stock is traded.

**Net Return:** The total yield after taxes (and/or inflation) earned by the investment.

**New Issue:** A stock or bond sold by a corporation for the first time. Proceeds may be issued to retire outstanding securities of the company, for new plant or equipment, for additional working capital, or to go to a selling shareholder.

**Noncancelable:** Policies that may not be canceled (during a specified term) by the insurer, but the term *non-can* should not be applied to disability or health policies unless they are also guaranteed renewable.

**Nonqualified Retirement Plan:** A retirement plan that is not regulated by a government agency like the IRS, DOL, etc. These plans, normally sold by commission insurance agents, are frequently very inefficient due to high commissions. They purport to have the following benefits: (1) privacy, (2) no maximum contributions, (3) no tax on gains due to the insurance policies' tax-deferred status, (4) no tax on withdrawals due to using "loan" provisions, and (5) possible estate tax benefits. Beware of nonqualified retirement plans suggested by commission advisors or fee and commission advisors.

**Normal Retirement Age:** The time when a participant attains retirement age under a plan. Usually, it is age sixty-five; however, it may be another age (as set forth in the plan) and may also require a stated period of plan participants. Full vesting is required when a participant attains normal retirement age.

**Odd Lot:** An amount of stock less than the established hundred-share unit or ten-share unit of trading.

**No-Load Fund:** A mutual fund that charges no sales fee to buy and no sales fee to sell. No-load funds are usually the best to buy due to their low costs and professional management. (See also: **Load, Front-End Load,** and **Back-End Load**)

**Open-End Investment Company:** By definition under the 1940 Act, an investment company (mutual funds) that has outstanding redeemable shares. Also generally applied to those investment companies like mutual funds, which continuously offer new shares to the public and stand ready at any time to redeem their outstanding shares.

**Open-End Mutual Fund:** A mutual fund that allows investors to buy shares directly from the mutual fund company and stands ready to redeem shares whenever shareholders are ready to sell. Open-end funds may issue new shares any time there is a demand for more shares from investors. Shareholders buy and sell shares at the fund's net asset value (plus a possible sales fee), in contrast to a closed-end mutual fund, which trades like stock on a stock exchange. Rather than selling at net asset value, closed-end fund shares trade at whatever price the market is willing to pay.

**Option:** A right to buy or sell specific securities or properties at a specified price within a specified time.

**Ordinary Life Insurance:** Also known as *straight life* or *whole life*. Premiums are computed to be paid for life.

**Overbought:** An opinion as to volume and its relationship to price levels. May refer to a security that has had a sharp rise or to the market as a whole after a period of vigorous buying which, at least in the short term, has left prices too high (used as a signal to sell).

**Oversold:** The reverse of overbought. A single security or a market that has declined to an unreasonable level (used as a signal to buy).

**Over-the-Counter:** A market for investments made up of securities dealers who may or may not be members of a securities exchange. Over-the-counter is mainly a market made electronically and over the telephone. Thousands of companies have insufficient shares outstanding, stockholders, or earnings to warrant application for listing on a major (NYSE) exchange. Securities of these companies are traded in the over-the-counter market between dealers who act either as principals (ie, represent themselves) or as brokers for customers.

**Paper Profit:** An unrealized profit on an unsold investment. Paper profits become realized profits when the security is sold.

**Partnership:** A partnership is usually a contract of two or more persons to unite their property, labor, or skill, or some of them, to share the profits and risks.

**PBGC:** Pension Benefit Guarantee Corporation.

**Penny Stocks:** Low-priced issues, often highly speculative, selling at less than $1 to $5 a share. Frequently used as a term of disparagement, although a few penny stocks have developed into investment-caliber issues. Many international companies have low-priced stocks due to the customs of their markets.

**Pension Plan:** A qualified retirement plan established by an employer for its employees, including profit-sharing plans, stock bonus plans, thrift plans, target benefit plans, money purchase plans, defined benefit plans, and employee stock ownership plans.

**Plan Administrator:** The person designated by the plan documentation as administrator. If no designation is made, the plan administrator is the employer. The plan administrator is the person responsible for managing the day-to-day affairs of the plan.

**Plan Participant:** An employee who has met the age, service, or other requirements of his or her employer's retirement plan.

**Point:** In the case of stock, a point means $1. If ABC shares rise three points, each share has risen $3. With bonds, a point means $10. A bond is quoted as a percentage of $1,000. In the case of market averages, the word *point* means merely that. If, for example, the Dow-Jones Industrial Average rises from 10870 to 10871, it has risen a point. A point in this average is not equivalent to $1.

**Pooled Income Fund:** A type of annuity that pools the assets of a number of people, each sharing the income in proportion to their ownership.

**Portfolio:** Holdings of securities by an individual or institution. A portfolio may contain international and domestic bonds and stocks. A portfolio is usually constructed around an investment philosophy to achieve specific goals. A bunch of investments doesn't necessarily mean a portfolio.

**Preferred Stock:** A senior class of stock with a claim on the company's earnings before payment may be made on the common stock and usually entitled to priority over common stock if the company liquidates. It is usually entitled to dividends at a specified rate when declared by the board of directors, depending on the terms of the issue.

**Premium:** The amount by which a preferred stock or bond may sell above its par value. In the case of a new issue of bonds or stocks, premium is the amount the market price rises over the original selling price.

**Price-Earnings Ratio (P/E):** The price of a share of common stock divided by its earnings per share for a twelve-month period. P/E is Wall Street's most commonly used ratio to determine a stock's value to investors. A company with a stock price of $20 and earnings per share of $1 has a 20 P/E ($20 divided by $1), while a company with a stock price of $10 and the same $1 in earnings per share has a 10 P/E. The higher a stock's P/E, the more expensive the stock is relative to its earnings.

**Price-NAV Ratio (P/NAV):** The market price of a closed-end fund divided by its net asset value (NAV). P/NAV serves as a valuation indicator. Closed-end funds selling at a *discount* will have P/NAV ratios below 100 percent; those at a *premium* will have P/NAV ratios in excess of 100 percent.

**Profit-Sharing Plan:** A type of defined contribution retirement plan whereby employers have the right, but not the obligation, to make contributions (not to exceed 15 percent of wages) to eligible employees each year.

**Property and Casualty Insurance:** Insurance coverage to provide for the replacement of or compensation for property lost, stolen, damaged, or destroyed, etc.

**Prospectus:** The document containing important information that offers a new issue or continuously issued securities like mutual funds to the public. It is required under the Securities Act of 1933.

**Proxy:** Written authorization given by a shareholder to someone else to represent him or her and vote his or her shares at a shareholders' meeting.

**Proxy Statement:** Important information required by the SEC to be given to stockholders as a prerequisite to solicitation of proxies for a security, subject to the requirements of Securities Exchange Act.

**Prudent-Man Rule:** The standard under which a fiduciary must act. The fiduciary is required to act "with the care, skill, prudence, and diligence under the circumstances then prevailing that a prudent man acting in a like capacity and familiar with such matters would use in the conduct of an enterprise of a like character and with like aims." This general rule requires a retirement plan fiduciary to exercise "care, skill, and prudence" in relation to the investment assets in a qualified retirement plan.

**Put:** An option to sell a specified number of shares at a specified price within a specified period of time. The opposite of a call.

**QDRO:** Qualified Domestic Relations Order (See **Qualified Domestic Relations Order**).

**QPA:** Qualified Pension Accountant (pension plans).

**Qualified Domestic Relations Order (QDRO):** A court order issued under a state's domestic relations law that relates to the payment of child support or alimony, or to marital property rights. A QDRO creates or recognizes an alternate payee's right or assigns to an alternate payee the right to receive plan benefits payable to a participant. The alternate payee may be, for example, the participant's spouse, former spouse, or dependent.

**Qualified Pension Plan (Tax-Qualified Plan):** A plan that meets the requirements of the Internal Revenue Code, generally Section 401(a). The advantage of qualification is that the plan is eligible for special tax considerations. For example, employers are permitted to deduct contributions to the plan even though the benefits provided under the plan are deferred to a later date.

**Quotation:** Often shortened to *quote*. The highest bid to buy and the lowest offer to sell a security in a given market at a given time. If you ask your broker for a quote on a stock, she or he may come back with something like "20 1/2 to 21." This means that $20.50 is the highest price any buyer wanted to pay at the time the quote was given and that $21.00 was the lowest price any seller would take at the same time.

**Rally:** A quick rise in the general price level of the market or in an individual stock.

**Real Estate Investment Trust (REIT):** An equity trust that can hold real estate income and growth properties and offer shares that are publicly traded.

**Redemption Fee:** Sales fee or back-end load charged by some mutual funds to shareholders when they sell their shares. Redemption fees are a bad deal if they originate because of commissions. Funds with redemption fees usually have higher expenses than true no-load, no-commission funds. (See **Back-End Load**)

**Red Herring:** A preliminary prospectus used to obtain indications of interest from prospective buyers of a new issue of stock.

**Registered Representative:** Usually a full-time employee of a broker who has met the requirements of an exchange as to background and knowledge of the securities business.

**Reinvestment Risk:** One of the risks facing holders of fixed-income securities like bonds and CDs during periods of falling interest rates. The risk is that the investor will be forced to reinvest interest or principal payments at lower interest rates. For example, if you have a maturing CD that had a relatively high interest rate, you are forced to reinvest at a lower rate if interest rates have fallen.

**Return:** Another term for yield.

**Reverse Mortgage:** A financing arrangement for older homeowners to use their equity to remain in their homes. The homeowner borrows from a lending institution an amount equal to 60 percent to 80 percent of the home value, and the institution pays out the loan funds monthly for a certain period. At the end of the loan period, the homeowner has to repay the loan, usually by sale of the home. If the homeowner dies before the end of the loan payment period, the house is sold to satisfy the debt. "Private" reverse mortgages between well-off children and their parents are useful tools to help parents stay in their home.

**RIA:** Registered Investment Advisor (investment, money management). An advisor registered with the SEC to give investment advice.

**Rights:** When a company wants to raise more funds by issuing additional securities, it may give its stockholders the opportunity, ahead of others, to buy the new securities in proportion to the number of shares each owns. The piece of paper evidencing this privilege is called a right. Because the additional stock is usually offered to stockholders below the current market price, rights ordinarily have a market value of their own and are actively traded. In most cases, they must be exercised within a relatively short period of time. Failure to exercise or sell rights may result in actual loss to the holder.

**Rollover:** A method of avoiding the substantial tax bite of a lump sum retirement plan payment, allowing it to be rolled over into an IRA or similar vehicle to continue its deferred tax status. Certain payouts from pension plans may also be rolled over to an IRA or to another employer's plan.

**Rollover IRA Account:** An individual retirement account (IRA) that is established to receive a distribution from a qualified plan so that the income tax on the distribution will be deferred.

**Round Lot:** A unit of trading or a multiple thereof. On most US exchanges, the unit of trading is one hundred shares in the case of stocks and $1,000 par value in the case of bonds. In some inactive stocks, the unit of trading is ten shares. Global exchanges may have round lots of between one and ten thousand shares.

**Rule of 72:** A rough financial formula for calculating the amount of time it takes an investment to double at any rate of return. Divide the rate of return into 72.

**Segregated Account:** A separate subaccount within a retirement plan trust consisting of only one plan participant's account balance and not affected by the investment performance of the rest of the plan investments.

**SAR/SEP:** Salary Reduction/Simplified Employee Pension Plan. A type of IRA similar to a 40lk.

**Selling Short:** Selling stock not owned. A risky technique of borrowing stock in anticipation of a drop in stock value that will bring rewards. Instead of looking for market winners, the short seller looks for losers. Short selling can also be used to hedge a portfolio.

**Simplified Employee Pension Plan (SEP):** A retirement program that takes the form of individual retirement accounts for all eligible employees (subject to special rules on contributions and eligibility).

**Socially Conscious Investor:** An investor who allows her or his values and/or religious philosophy to influence her or his investing. Avoiding tobacco, alcohol, arms makers, polluters, etc, is one way these investors exercise their might. Another is to invest in companies that "do good," like having good employee relations, women in management, etc.

**Social Mutual Funds:** Mutual funds that are driven not just by profit potential but also by principles and values.

**Speculator:** One who is willing to assume a relatively large risk in the hope of gain. Her or his principal concern is to increase her or his capital rather than predictable dividend income. The speculator may buy and sell the same day or speculate in an enterprise she or he does not expect to be profitable for years.

**Split:** The division of the outstanding shares of a company into a larger number of shares. A 3-for-1 split by a company with 1 million shares currently outstanding results in 3 million shares outstanding after the split. Each holder of one hundred shares before the 3-to-1 split would have three hundred shares, although proportionate equity in the company would remain the same; one hundred parts of 1 million are the equivalent of three hundred parts of 3 million, etc. Stock splits make a company's stock easier to trade by keeping its stock price lower than it would be without the split, thus making it less costly to buy a round lot of shares.

**Sponsor:** Employer/company that elects to establish a qualified retirement plan and be responsible for the cost of funding and maintaining the retirement trust with contributions and the payment of expenses.

**Spousal IRA:** An IRA that is established for the nonworking spouse of an employee who qualified for an IRA. A contribution of $2,250, instead of $2,000, is permitted, but the maximum contribution for either spouse is $2,000.

**Spread:** The difference between the bid price and the offering price.

**Stock Bonus Plan:** A defined contribution retirement plan that is similar to a profit-sharing plan except that the employer's contributions do not have to be made out of profits, and benefit payments generally must be made in employer company stock.

**Street Name:** Securities held under strict guidelines in the name of a broker instead of the customer's name are said to be carried in a street name account. This occurs when the securities have been bought on margin or when the customer wishes, for convenience and security, to have the security held by a broker.

**Subchapter "S" Corporation:** Business with a legal corporate form that pays income taxes like a sole proprietor.

**Suitability Rule:** The rule of fair practice that requires an investment seller to have reasonable grounds for believing that a recommendation to a customer is suitable on the basis of the person's financial objectives, risk tolerance, net worth, and abilities.

**Summary Annual Report:** A summary of the financial activity within a qualified plan on any given plan year, which each plan participant is required to receive.

**Summary Plan Description (SPD):** A detailed, but hopefully easily understood, document describing a pension plan's provisions that must be provided to participants and plan beneficiaries.

**Target Benefit Plan:** A cross between a defined benefit plan and a money purchase retirement plan. Similar to a defined benefit plan in that the annual contribution is determined by the amount needed each year to accumulate a fund sufficient to pay a targeted retirement benefit to each participant on reaching retirement. Similar to a money purchase plan in that contributions are allocated to separate accounts maintained for each participant. (See also: **Defined Benefit Plan** and **Money Purchase Pension Plan**)

**Tax-Deductible:** Expenses and items that are able to reduce the amount of taxable income. Examples include medical expenses, IRA contributions, charitable deductions, and interest paid.

**Tax Deferral:** A method that defers the payment of taxes on income until a future time. The rationale is that future tax brackets will be lower, enabling one to compound the tax savings, while the payment of the tax will be made with inflated dollars.

**Tax Incentive:** Corporate or venture vehicle that includes major tax incentives to invest.

**Tax-Sheltered Investment:** An investment that has an expectation of economic profit, made even more attractive because of the timing of the profit or the way it is taxed, generally having some or all of the following characteristics: (*a*) capital gains opportunities; (*b*) high deductions; (*c*) deferral of income; (*d*) depletion; (*e*) accelerated depreciation; (*f*) leverage. The flow-through of tax benefits is a material factor, regardless of whether the entity is organized as a *private program* or a *public program*. Common forms of tax-sheltered investments include cattle breeding, cattle feeding, equipment leasing, oil and gas, and real estate.

**Tax Shelter Plan:** A slang term used to describe a qualified retirement plan that has been established for the benefit of the owner or specific officers.

**Tender Offer:** An offer to buy securities at a specific price. Can be used by a closed-end fund or company to buy back some of its shares because it feels shares are at bargain levels. Tender offers can also be used by raiders to try to acquire shares of a target company.

**Time Diversification:** The idea that the longer securities are held, the lower their risk since good market periods are averaged in with bad ones.

**Time-Sharing:** A creative real estate financing technique that allows the use of property on a time-shared basis, while building equity for all of the owners. There are two types: right-to-use (membership right) and interval ownership (purchase of a particular week or weeks each year).

**Top Down:** An investment strategy where the investor looks at broad economic trends to find which types of investments appear to be best positioned for growth, and then selects individual investments based on that economic assessment. It is the opposite of a bottom-up strategy, in which an investor assesses an individual investment strictly on its own merits, irrespective of the overall economy. (See also: **Bottom Up**)

**TPA:** Third-Party Administrator (employee benefits).

**Trader:** One who buys and sells for his own account for short-term profit.

**Treasury Bills (T-Bills):** Short-term US government investments with no stated interest rate, sold at a discount with competitive bidding. For example, a Treasury bill may be sold at $9,500 with a value at maturity of $10,000 in one year.

**Treasury Bonds:** Government bonds issued in $1,000 units with a maturity of five years or longer. They are traded on the market like other bonds.

**Treasury Notes:** Government bonds, not legally restricted as to interest rates, with maturities of from one to five years.

**Treasury Stock:** Stock issued by a company but later reacquired. It may be held in the company's treasury indefinitely, reissued to the public, or retired. Treasury stock receives no dividends and has no vote while held by the company.

**Trust:** A fund established under local trust law to hold and administer the assets of a plan.

**Trustee:** Individual or entity that assumes responsibility to safeguard the assets of the retirement trust for the benefit of the plan participants.

**Trustees:** The parties named in the trust instrument or plan authorized to hold the assets of the plan for the benefit of the participants. The trustees may function merely in the capacity of custodian of the assets, or they may also be given authority over the investment of the assets. Their function is determined by the trust instrument or, if no separate trust agreement is executed, under the trust provisions of the plan.

**TSA:** Tax-Sheltered Annuity. 403(b) retirement plan available to employees of some schools, hospitals, and other charities.

**12b-1 Fee:** A modest to very large fee assessed annually by some mutual funds to cover advertising, sales, and marketing expenses. The fee is deducted directly from each shareholder's holdings, reduces its return by that amount, and usually represents .25 percent to less than 1 percent of net asset value. 12b-1 fees can up to double a fund's expenses. Beware of these fees.

**Umbrella Liability:** Insurance coverage in excess of underlying liability policies; provides coverage for many situations excluded by underlying policies and may also include excess major medical expense coverage.

**Unlisted:** A security not listed on a stock exchange.

**Value Investing:** An investment philosophy that places primary emphasis on finding bargains through price as opposed to forecasted earnings growth. Value investors look for solid companies with good prospects at bargain prices and closed-end funds at attractive discounts.

**Variable Annuity:** An annuity that has the (possible) benefits of higher yield by allowing the annuitant to invest in mutual fund–type portfolios (stocks, bonds, etc).

**Variable Rate Mortgage:** A financing technique in real estate that allows the interest charged on the mortgage to fluctuate with the rise and fall of market interest rates.

**Vested Benefits:** Accrued benefits of a participant that have become nonforfeitable under the vesting schedule adopted by the plan. Thus, for example, if the schedule provided for vesting at the rate of 10 percent per year, a participant who has been credited with six years of service has a right to 60 percent of his or her accrued benefit. If he or she terminates his or her service without being credited with any additional years of service, he or she is entitled to receive 60 percent of his or her accrued benefits.

**Vesting:** The nonforfeitable right that a participant has in her or his account balance of a qualified retirement plan trust. This right is accrued based on the number of hours the participant works for the sponsor for a given number of years.

**Voting Right:** The stockholder's right to vote his or her stock in the affairs of his or her company. Most common shares have one vote each. Preferred stock usually has the right to vote when preferred dividends are in default for a specified period. The right to vote may be delegated by the stockholder to another person.

**Warrant:** A certificate giving the holder the right to purchase securities at a stipulated price within a specified time limit or perpetually. Sometimes a warrant is offered with securities as an inducement to buy.

**When Issued:** A short form of "when, as, and if issued." The term indicates a conditional transaction in a security authorized for issuance but not yet actually issued. All "when issued" transactions are on an "if" basis, to be settled if and when the actual security is issued and the exchange or National Association of Securities Dealers rules that the transactions are to be settled.

**Yield:** Also known as income return. The (usually annual) dividends or interest paid by a company expressed as a percentage of the current price. A stock with a current market value of $20 a share that has paid $1 in dividends in the preceding twelve months is said to return 5 percent ($1.00/$20.00). The current return on a bond or other investment is figured the same way.

**Yield to Maturity:** The total return that would be realized if a bond were purchased at its present price and held to maturity or "call." In order to earn the yield to maturity, the investor must also reinvest all interest payments at a rate equal to the yield to maturity. This also assumes that the issuer will make all promised payments on time and in full.

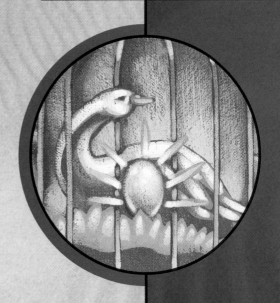

# Investor Resources

## Worksheet
# Aggressive Portfolio

**3% yields, 35% volatility
6-year time frame**

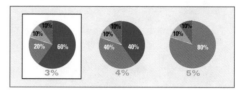

Portfolio Registration _____

Custodial Broker _____

Phone Number _____

Account Number _____

| | Approximate Percentage | Amount Invested | Date |
|---|---|---|---|
| **60% Balanced Funds** | | | |
| 1. _____ | % | | |
| 2. _____ | % | | |
| 3. _____ | % | | |
| 4. _____ | % | | |
| 5. _____ | % | | |
| 6. _____ | % | | |
| **20% Stock Funds** | | | |
| 1. _____ | % | | |
| 2. _____ | % | | |
| 3. _____ | % | | |
| 4. _____ | % | | |
| **No bond funds, no money market funds** | | | |
| **10% Gold and Natural Resource Funds** | | | |
| 1. _____ | % | | |
| 2. _____ | % | | |
| **10% International Stock Funds** | | | |
| 1. _____ | % | | |
| 2. _____ | % | | |

**Notes** _____

## Worksheet

# Growth Portfolio

**3% yields, 30% volatility
5-year time frame**

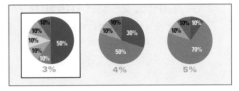

Portfolio Registration  _____

Custodial Broker  _____

Phone Number  _____

Account Number  _____

| | Approximate Percentage | Amount Invested | Date |
|---|---|---|---|
| **50% Balanced Funds** | | | |
| 1. _____ | % | | |
| 2. _____ | % | | |
| 3. _____ | % | | |
| **10% Stock Funds** | | | |
| 1. _____ | % | | |
| 2. _____ | % | | |
| **10% Bond Funds** | | | |
| 1. _____ | % | | |
| 2. _____ | % | | |
| **10% Money Market Funds** | | | |
| 1. _____ | % | | |
| **10% Gold and Natural Resource Funds** | | | |
| 1. _____ | % | | |
| 2. _____ | % | | |
| **10% International Stock Funds** | | | |
| 1. _____ | % | | |
| 2. _____ | % | | |

**Notes**  _____

## Worksheet
# Balanced Portfolio

**3% yields, 25% volatility
5-year time frame**

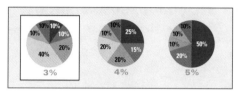

Portfolio Registration  _____

Custodial Broker  _____

Phone Number  _____

Account Number  _____

| | Approximate Percentage | Amount Invested | Date |
|---|---|---|---|
| **10% Balanced Funds** | | | |
| 1. _____ | % | | |
| 2. _____ | % | | |
| **10% Stock Funds** | | | |
| 1. _____ | % | | |
| 2. _____ | % | | |
| **20% Bond Funds** | | | |
| 1. _____ | % | | |
| 2. _____ | % | | |
| 3. _____ | % | | |
| **40% Money Market Funds** | | | |
| 1. _____ | % | | |
| **10% Gold and Natural Resource Funds** | | | |
| 1. _____ | % | | |
| 2. _____ | % | | |
| **10% International Stock Funds** | | | |
| 1. _____ | % | | |
| 2. _____ | % | | |

**Notes**
_____

**Worksheet**

# Yield Portfolio

**3% yields, 15% volatility**
**4-year time frame**

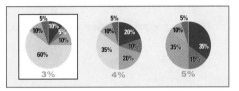

Portfolio Registration  _____

Custodial Broker  _____

Phone Number  _____

Account Number  _____

| | Approximate Percentage | Amount Invested | Date |
|---|---|---|---|
| **10% Balanced Funds** | | | |
| 1. _____ | % | | |
| 2. _____ | % | | |
| **5% Stock Funds** | | | |
| 1. _____ | % | | |
| 2. _____ | % | | |
| **10% Bond Funds** | | | |
| 1. _____ | % | | |
| 2. _____ | % | | |
| 3. _____ | % | | |
| **60% Money Market Funds** | | | |
| 1. _____ | % | | |
| **10% Gold and Natural Resource Funds** | | | |
| 1. _____ | % | | |
| 2. _____ | % | | |
| **5% International Stock Funds** | | | |
| 1. _____ | % | | |
| 2. _____ | % | | |

**Notes**
_____

**Worksheet**

# Capital Preservation Portfolio

**3% yields, 5% volatility**
**1-year time frame**

Portfolio Registration _____

Custodial Broker _____

Phone Number _____

Account Number _____

| | Approximate Percentage | Amount Invested | Date |
|---|---|---|---|
| **5% Balanced Funds** | | | |
| 1. _____ | % | | |
| 2. _____ | % | | |
| 3. _____ | % | | |
| **No stock funds** | | | |
| **5% Bond Funds** | | | |
| 1. _____ | % | | |
| 2. _____ | % | | |
| 3. _____ | % | | |
| **80% Money Market Funds** | | | |
| 1. _____ | % | | |
| **5% Gold and Natural Resource Funds** | | | |
| 1. _____ | % | | |
| 2. _____ | % | | |
| 3. _____ | % | | |
| **5% International Stock Funds** | | | |
| 1. _____ | % | | |
| 2. _____ | % | | |

**Notes**

## Worksheet

# Aggressive Portfolio

**4% yields, 35% volatility**
**6-year time frame**

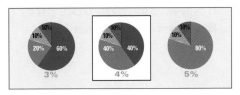

| Portfolio Registration | |
|---|---|
| Custodial Broker | |
| Phone Number | |
| Account Number | |

| | Approximate Percentage | Amount Invested | Date |
|---|---|---|---|
| **40% Balanced Funds** | | | |
| 1. | % | | |
| 2. | % | | |
| 3. | % | | |
| 4. | % | | |
| **40% Stock Funds** | | | |
| 1. | % | | |
| 2. | % | | |
| 3. | % | | |
| 4. | % | | |
| **No bond funds, no money market funds** | | | |
| **10% Gold and Natural Resource Funds** | | | |
| 1. | % | | |
| 2. | % | | |
| 3. | % | | |
| **10% International Stock Funds** | | | |
| 1. | % | | |
| 2. | % | | |
| 3. | % | | |

**Notes**

## Worksheet

# Growth Portfolio

**4% yields, 30% volatility**
**5-year time frame**

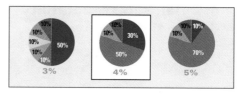

Portfolio Registration _____

Custodial Broker _____

Phone Number _____

Account Number _____

| | Approximate Percentage | Amount Invested | Date |
|---|---|---|---|
| **30% Balanced Funds** | | | |
| 1. _____ | % | | |
| 2. _____ | % | | |
| 3. _____ | % | | |
| 4. _____ | % | | |
| **50% Stock Funds** | | | |
| 1. _____ | % | | |
| 2. _____ | % | | |
| 3. _____ | % | | |
| 4. _____ | % | | |
| 5. _____ | % | | |
| 6. _____ | % | | |
| **No bond funds, no money market funds** | | | |
| **10% Gold and Natural Resource Funds** | | | |
| 1. _____ | % | | |
| 2. _____ | % | | |
| **10% International Stock Funds** | | | |
| 1. _____ | % | | |
| 2. _____ | % | | |

**Notes** _____

**Worksheet**

# Balanced Portfolio

**4% yields, 25% volatility**
**5-year time frame**

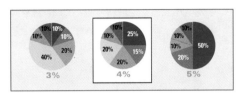

Portfolio Registration  _____
Custodial Broker  _____
Phone Number  _____
Account Number  _____

|  | Approximate Percentage | Amount Invested | Date |
|---|---|---|---|
| **25% Balanced Funds** |  |  |  |
| 1. _____ | % |  |  |
| 2. _____ | % |  |  |
| 3. _____ | % |  |  |
| 4. _____ | % |  |  |
| **15% Stock Funds** |  |  |  |
| 1. _____ | % |  |  |
| 2. _____ | % |  |  |
| **20% Bond Funds** |  |  |  |
| 1. _____ | % |  |  |
| 2. _____ | % |  |  |
| **20% Money Market Funds** |  |  |  |
| 1. _____ | % |  |  |
| 2. _____ | % |  |  |
| **10% Gold and Natural Resource Funds** |  |  |  |
| 1. _____ | % |  |  |
| **5% International Stock Funds** |  |  |  |
| 1. _____ | % |  |  |

**Notes** _____

## Worksheet
# Yield Portfolio

**4% yields, 15% volatility**
**4-year time frame**

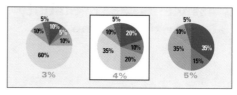

Portfolio Registration _____

Custodial Broker _____

Phone Number _____

Account Number _____

| | Approximate Percentage | Amount Invested | Date |
|---|---|---|---|
| **20% Balanced Funds** | | | |
| 1. _____ | % | | |
| 2. _____ | % | | |
| 3. _____ | % | | |
| **10% Stock Funds** | | | |
| 1. _____ | % | | |
| 2. _____ | % | | |
| **20% Bond Funds** | | | |
| 1. _____ | % | | |
| 2. _____ | % | | |
| 3. _____ | % | | |
| **35% Money Market Funds** | | | |
| 1. _____ | % | | |
| **10% Gold and Natural Resource Funds** | | | |
| 1. _____ | % | | |
| 2. _____ | % | | |
| **5% International Stock Funds** | | | |
| 1. _____ | % | | |

**Notes**

**Worksheet**

# Capital Preservation Portfolio

**4% yields, 5% volatility
1-year time frame**

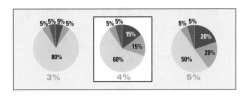

Portfolio Registration _____
Custodial Broker _____
Phone Number _____
Account Number _____

| | Approximate Percentage | Amount Invested | Date |
|---|---|---|---|
| **15% Balanced Funds** | | | |
| 1. _____ | % | | |
| 2. _____ | % | | |
| 3. _____ | % | | |
| 4. _____ | % | | |
| **No stock funds** | | | |
| **15% Bond Funds** | | | |
| 1. _____ | % | | |
| 2. _____ | % | | |
| 3. _____ | % | | |
| **60% Money Market Funds** | | | |
| 1. _____ | % | | |
| **5% Gold and Natural Resource Funds** | | | |
| 1. _____ | % | | |
| 2. _____ | % | | |
| **5% International Stock Funds** | | | |
| 1. _____ | % | | |
| 2. _____ | % | | |

**Notes**

## Worksheet
# Aggressive Portfolio

**5% yields, 35% volatility**
**6-year time frame**

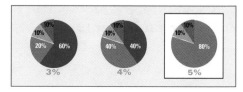

Portfolio Registration _____
Custodial Broker _____
Phone Number _____
Account Number _____

| | Approximate Percentage | Amount Invested | Date |
|---|---|---|---|
| **80% Balanced Funds** | | | |
| 1. _____ | % | | |
| 2. _____ | % | | |
| 3. _____ | % | | |
| 4. _____ | % | | |
| 5. _____ | % | | |
| 6. _____ | % | | |
| 7. _____ | % | | |
| **No bond funds, no money market funds** | | | |
| **10% Gold and Natural Resource Funds** | | | |
| 1. _____ | % | | |
| 2. _____ | % | | |
| 3. _____ | % | | |
| **10% International Stock Funds** | | | |
| 1. _____ | % | | |
| 2. _____ | % | | |
| 3. _____ | % | | |

**Notes** _____

**Worksheet**
# Growth Portfolio

## 5% yields, 30% volatility
## 5-year time frame

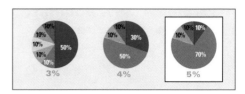

Portfolio Registration  _____

Custodial Broker  _____

Phone Number  _____

Account Number  _____

| | Approximate Percentage | Amount Invested | Date |
|---|---|---|---|
| **10% Balanced Funds** | | | |
| 1. _____ | % | | |
| 2. _____ | % | | |
| 3. _____ | % | | |
| **70% Stock Funds** | | | |
| 1. _____ | % | | |
| 2. _____ | % | | |
| 3. _____ | % | | |
| 4. _____ | % | | |
| 5. _____ | % | | |
| 6. _____ | % | | |
| 7. _____ | % | | |
| **No bond funds, no money market funds** | | | |
| **10% Gold and Natural Resource Funds** | | | |
| 1. _____ | % | | |
| 2. _____ | % | | |
| **10% International Stock Funds** | | | |
| 1. _____ | % | | |
| 2. _____ | % | | |

**Notes**

## Worksheet
# Balanced Portfolio

**5% yields, 25% volatility
5-year time frame**

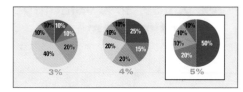

Portfolio Registration _____

Custodial Broker _____

Phone Number _____

Account Number _____

| | Approximate Percentage | Amount Invested | Date |
|---|---|---|---|
| **50% Balanced Funds** | | | |
| 1. _____ | % | | |
| 2. _____ | % | | |
| 3. _____ | % | | |
| 4. _____ | % | | |
| **20% Stock Funds** | | | |
| 1. _____ | % | | |
| 2. _____ | % | | |
| **10% Bond Funds** | | | |
| 1. _____ | % | | |
| 2. _____ | % | | |
| **No money market funds** | | | |
| **10% Gold and Natural Resource Funds** | | | |
| 1. _____ | % | | |
| 2. _____ | % | | |
| **10% International Stock Funds** | | | |
| 1. _____ | % | | |
| 2. _____ | % | | |

**Notes** _____

## Worksheet
# Yield Portfolio

**5% yields, 15% volatility
4-year time frame**

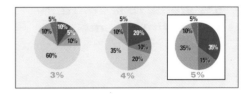

Portfolio Registration _____
Custodial Broker _____
Phone Number _____
Account Number _____

| | Approximate Percentage | Amount Invested | Date |
|---|---|---|---|
| **35% Balanced Funds** | | | |
| 1. _____ | % | | |
| 2. _____ | % | | |
| 3. _____ | % | | |
| | | | |
| **15% Stock Funds** | | | |
| 1. _____ | % | | |
| 2. _____ | % | | |
| | | | |
| **35% Bond Funds** | | | |
| 1. _____ | % | | |
| 2. _____ | % | | |
| 3. _____ | % | | |
| | | | |
| **No money market funds** | | | |
| | | | |
| **10% Gold and Natural Resource Funds** | | | |
| 1. _____ | % | | |
| 2. _____ | % | | |
| | | | |
| **5% International Stock Funds** | | | |
| 1. _____ | % | | |
| 2. _____ | % | | |

**Notes**

## Worksheet
# Capital Preservation Portfolio

**5% yields, 5% volatility**
**1-year time frame**

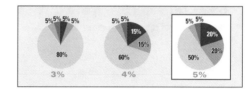

Portfolio Registration  _____

Custodial Broker  _____

Phone Number  _____

Account Number  _____

| | Approximate Percentage | Amount Invested | Date |
|---|---|---|---|
| **20% Balanced Funds** | | | |
| 1. _____ | % | | |
| 2. _____ | % | | |
| 3. _____ | % | | |
| 4. _____ | % | | |
| | | | |
| **No stock funds** | | | |
| | | | |
| **20% Bond Funds** | | | |
| 1. _____ | % | | |
| 2. _____ | % | | |
| 3. _____ | % | | |
| | | | |
| **50% Money Market Funds** | | | |
| 1. _____ | % | | |
| | | | |
| **5% Gold and Natural Resource Funds** | | | |
| 1. _____ | % | | |
| 2. _____ | % | | |
| | | | |
| **5% International Stock Funds** | | | |
| 1. _____ | % | | |
| 2. _____ | % | | |

**Notes**  _____

# index

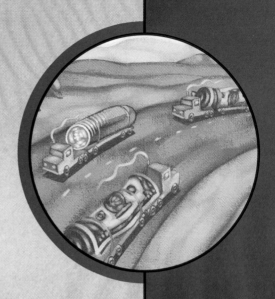

# A

Age-weighted retirement plans, 65
American Express Financial Direct
(discount broker), 105
Ameritrade (discount broker), 105
APT. *See* Asset protection trusts
(APTs)
Asset protection planning, 35
Asset protection trusts (APTs), 35–36
Assets and liabilities worksheet, 13–15
Assisted living care, investment
considerations for, 130

# B

Banking, four Cs of, 22
Bear markets, retirement portfolios
and, 118–120
Benefit guaranteed plans, 4
Bond funds, 97
Bonds, 5
Brokers, stock
discount, 90–91, 103–105
selecting, 90–91
Budgets
calculating monthly, 18
worksheets for, 19

# C

Cash management accounts (CMAs),
92
Charles Schwab (discount broker), 103
Contracts, 32, 34
Cooking schools, 62
Cruise lines, 124

# D

Debt, 4–5
investments and, 20–22
managing, 20
ten rules for managing, 22–24
worksheet for restructuring of, for
new physicians, 21

# Defined benefit plans (DBPs), 65–66
Disability income insurance, 28
worksheet for, 32, 33
Discount brokers, 90–91, 103–105
Dispositions, event-driven, 145–147
Dividends, retirement portfolios and,
118
Dividend yields, 74–75
for measuring stock market cycles,
82
DLJ Direct (discount broker), 105
Dollar-cost-averaging, 108–110
sample portfolios, 110–115
Dream vacations, planning, 5
Durable power of attorney, 143

# E

Estate planning, 144–145
checklist for, 146
event-driven dispositions and,
145–147
E*Trade (discount broker), 104
Event-driven dispositions, 145–147

# F

Family limited partnerships (FLPs), 35
Fidelity (discount broker), 103
Financial management accounts, 92
FLP. *See* Family limited partnerships
(FLPs)
Four Cs of banking, 22
401k plans, 63
Future values
for lump sump of $1, 52–53
for $1 per year invested, 54–55

# G

Goals, investment, 86
Goals, retirement, 6
Gold funds, 97

## H

Health care needs, 4

## I

Income needs
    including Social Security in, 4
    quantifying, 3
Insurance. *See also* specific type of
        insurance
    key contract provisions for, 31–32
    monthly budget allotments for, 4
    retirement plans and, 26–27
International stock funds, 96
Investments. *See also* Portfolios,
        retirement
    anxiety and, 122
    controlling costs of, 90–91
    debt and, 20–22
    do-it-yourself strategy for, 87–90
    goal of, 86
    hiring professionals for, 122–123
    management fees, 80
    perception and reality of, 76, 79
    philosophy for, 77–78
    stocks, 72–74
IRAs, 58
    Roth, 40
Irrevocable trusts, 143

## J

Jack White (discount broker), 103
Job loss, 31

## L

Liabilities worksheet, 13–15
Liability insurance, 27
Life insurance, 28
    sample term rates for, 30
    worksheet for, 29
Long-term care, retirement planning
        and, 4

## M

Market cycle strategy, 84
Money market investments, 5
Money purchase plans, 61
Muriel Siebert (discount broker), 104
Mutual fund managers, selecting, 102
Mutual funds, 93–102
    tax implications of, 43

## N

National Discount Brokers, 104
Natural resources funds, 97

## O

Offshore trusts, 35–36

## P

Portfolios, retirement. *See also*
        Investments
    anxiety and, 122
    bear markets and, 118–120
    dividends and, 118
    do-it-yourself strategy for, 85
    goals for, 118
    hiring professionals for, 122–123
    long-term strategies for, 128–129
    management process for, 83
    managing, 82–84, 128–129
    obtaining income from, 118–121
    planning income from, 5–6
    risk tolerance and, 84
    volatility, 86
    worksheets for, 12
Postnuptial agreements, 27
Practices, selling, 47
Prenuptial agreements, 27
Probate, 142
Profit-sharing plans, 59–61
    age-weighted and new
            comparability, 65
Property insurance, 27

# R

Real estate investments, 5
Retirement
   debts and, 4–5
   insurance and, 26–27
   long-term care and, 4
   planning, 1–2
   quantifying income needs for, 3
   reality worksheet for, 51
   simple saving rules for, 48
   worksheet for, 7–11
Retirement enhancers, 4
Retirement income
   quantifying, 3
   Social Security and, 4
Retirement plans
   advisors for, 42
   age-weighted, 65
   comparison of, 67–68
   defined benefit plans, 65–66
   401k plans, 63
   IRAs, 58
   money purchase plans, 61
   new comparability profit-sharing
      plans, 65
   priority of funding, 38
   profit-sharing plans, 59–61
   SEPs, 59
   SIMPLE plans, 63–64
   tax benefits of, 38
   tax-qualified, 38–42
   tax-sheltered, 46–47
   worst mistakes regarding, 66–70
Retirement portfolios. *See* Portfolios,
   retirement
Revocable living trusts, 143
Risk tolerance, 86
   retirement portfolios and, 84
Roth IRAs, 40

# S

Saving, 46–47
   simple things to do for retirement,
      48
   ten percent rule of, 47–50
SEPs (Simplified Employee Pension)
   plans, 59
SIMPLE (Savings Incentive Match
   Plan for Employees) plans, 63–64
Social Security income, 4
Social values mutual funds, 98–100
Stock brokers
   discount, 90–91, 103–105
   selecting, 90–91
Stock funds, 95–96
Stock market, 5
   average annual returns, 88
   using dividends for measuring
      cycles, 82
Stocks, 72–74
   dividend yields of, 74–75
   as long-term investments, 86–87
   market returns for, 88

# T

Tax-qualified retirement plans, 38–42
Tax Sheltered 403(b) plans, 40
Tax-sheltered retirement plans,
   drawing on, 46–47
Ten percent rule of saving, 47–50
Travel, resources for, 137–138
Trusts, 143
   administration of, 144–145
TSAs. *See* Tax Sheltered 403(b) plans

# V

Vacations
   cooking schools for, 62
   cruise lines for, 124
   planning dream, 5
   resources for, 137–138
Vanguard (discount broker), 103
Volatility, retirement portfolios and, 86
Volunteerism, 136–140

# W

Wills, 142
Worksheets
    for aggressive portfolios, 170, 175,
        180
    for assets and liabilities, 13–15
    for balanced portfolios, 172, 177,
        182
    for capital preservation portfolios,
        174, 179, 184
    for debt restructuring—new
        physicians, 21
    for disability income insurance, 31,
        33
    for growth portfolios, 171, 176, 181
    for life insurance, 29
    for monthly budgets, 19
    for portfolios, 12
    for retirement, 7–11
    for retirement reality, 51
    for yield portfolios, 173, 178, 183

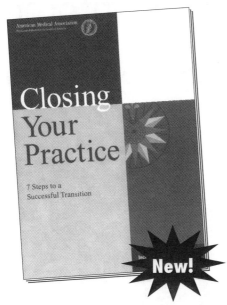

# Communicating health information over the Internet?

## Know Your Legal Risk!

The Internet offers health care providers enormous opportunity for sending and receiving health information quickly and easily. But with that opportunity also comes risk.

*Using The Internet for Health Information: Legal Issues,* new from the American Medical Association, will help you understand your legal risks and how to avoid or lessen them.

With expert advice from a knowledgeable health care attorney, you'll learn:

- Issues of medical/professional liability related to the patient-physician relationship

- Potential problems for Internet users related to state medical licensure and malpractice insurance coverage.

- Recommended steps to ensure confidentiality and privacy of Internet communications.

- How to use disclaimers to lower risk

**Lower your legal risk in Internet communications.**

Order your copy of *Using The Internet for Health Information: Legal Issues,* today!

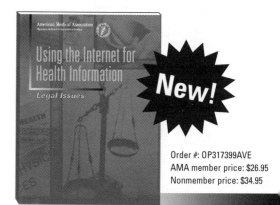

Order #: OP317399AVE
AMA member price: $26.95
Nonmember price: $34.95

## Order today toll free!
## 800 621-8335

**Use priority code: AVE** Visa, MasterCard, American Express, Optima accepted. Applicable state sales tax and shipping and handling added. Satisfaction guaranteed or return within 30 days for a full refund.

**Visit the AMA Web site at**
**www.ama-assn.org/catalog**

---

**AMA Information on Request Faxline**

Fast, easy access to complete product, service and ordering information. Call 800 621-8335, press 2, and follow the voice prompts. Information will arrive within a matter of minutes. Call anytime, 24 hours a day.

---

## American Medical Association
Physicians dedicated to the health of America